EDS SURVIVAL GUIDE

5 KEYS TO THRIVING WITH EHLERS-DANLOS SYNDROME

SONYA ZAPPONE

CONTENTS

Also by Sonya Zappone   v

Disclaimer   vii

The 5 A's of Thriving With EDS   xiii

Welcome Survivors and Thrivers!   xv

A Brief But Long History   1

KEY #1

First Things First   27

Awareness 101   34

Making Adjustments with Awareness   37

KEY #2

Needing Support   45

Adjusting to a New Reality   49

KEY #3

Acknowledgement   55

KEY #4

Action   63

KEY #5

Acceptance   71

BONUS #6

Accommodations   81

My Solutions List   85

7-DAY SELF-STARTER/SELF-LOVE CHECKLIST PLAN   87

CHALLENGE ACCEPTED?

DAY #1	91
DAY #2	93
DAY #3	95
DAY #4	97
DAY #5	99
DAY #6	101
DAY #7	103
From a Higher Perspective	105
Helpful Resources	107
About the Author	109

ALSO BY SONYA ZAPPONE

The Soul Doesn't Need a Million Dollars: 7 Secrets to Access Power Within You to Discover Purpose and Meaning in Work You Love

Connect to Soul: Poems for Yoga

DISCLAIMER
PLEASE READ BEFORE YOU BEGIN THIS BOOK

Firstly, I am not a mental health professional. This book is not a substitute for individual therapeutic care from a licensed professional. I encourage those who need emotional support to seek out therapy to meet individual needs and to get a correct (and accurate) diagnosis and treatment. If you are suffering from severe or debilitating anxiety or depression, this book is not a remedy, treatment, or cure. Please get the right support from your local agencies, clinics, and organizations that treat mental health issues.

This is my personal story, which includes insights, tips, and remedies that I have come up with over the years while dealing with my EDS. Chronic or severe conditions may need care and help from experienced clinicians. Please find adequate and additional resources for your needs. Although I am certified as a life coach, I am not a clinician. I do not hold any licenses to treat conditions like autism, Asperger's, depression, anxiety, adjustment disorders, etc. Always consult your physician before beginning any form of self-treatment. You may need more experienced, hands-on, and tailored help to get well. I will not be liable for any use or misuse of this information, as I am just a person sharing my helpful hints/tips in an educational manner.

Secondly, I am not a doctor. I do not have any medical training or expertise. I cannot diagnose, prescribe, or recommend any treatment for genetic disorders, including EDS. Also, I cannot advise any protocol to deal with EDS, Mast Cell Activation Syndrome (MCAS), Postural Orthostatic Tachycardia Syndrome (POTS), or any other disease or related condition. Please seek expert medical advice from doctors who specialize in your rare condition. Helpful resources and websites will be in the back of this book for you to seek out experts. Most importantly, always consult your doctor before beginning any form of exercise. Some forms of exercise can be harmful and are contraindicated for those with EDS. Be sure to know what to avoid. There are several things (certain exercises, hobbies, activities, medical treatment, medicines) it is best to refrain from. It is best/safest to have a physical therapist assisting and monitoring you at all times during exercise.

Furthermore, just because I have certain comorbidities such as MCAS doesn't mean that you have or will develop/sustain the conditions and injuries that I suffered. To date, there is no biomarker for hypermobile Ehlers-Danlos syndrome (hEDS), and so medical professionals cannot definitively diagnose my condition. My diagnosis has been based on clinical judgment of meeting the current criteria of physical observation and demonstration. Everyone is born with a unique set of genes. Additionally, not everyone with the same gene will have it expressed in exactly the same way. Conditions, vulnerabilities, and limitations may vary greatly. Outcomes vary, too. My life story and my childbirth history may or may not match what you or others with EDS experience. Keep in mind that every person's experience is different with EDS. Please take what is helpful and keep the knowledge as a database of wisdom from one woman with hEDS.

Lastly, I hope this book helps you in some way. Perhaps it will help to hear about someone else's struggles and experience with EDS so you feel less alone. May this book be a blessing to those who need validation on their healing journey. Please take my steps and the suggested **"Self-Reflections Questions"** as opportunities to do individual journal work to discover your own thoughts, feelings, experiences, reflections, and emotions. The **"My Solutions List"** is meant to show you alternative remedies that I used in conjunction with proper medical care, medicines, physician follow-up and therapeutic assessments. My **"7 Days of Self-**

Love and Self-Healing Section" is meant to show you what I did to get myself mentally and emotionally back on track toward helping myself. Many times my techniques helped me get to the right doctor. I did what's described in this book in conjunction with a life coach, therapist, doctor, geneticist, allergist, immunologist and other specialists following and treating my conditions. I do not suggest that self-help is the best, nor only form of help, but it certainly helped me.

Special Note: My *5 Keys to Thriving with EDS* is not required to survive or thrive with EDS. If you are reading this book, you are surviving your condition. Keep doing what works for you even if it's different from what I identified as key emotional steps. I encourage you to create your own blend of self-help strategies so that you can tailor *your* days with EDS to meet *your* needs and lifestyle. I urge you to use caution, common sense and logic. Be smart. Only you know what you are dealing with. Sometimes the doctors know more, sometimes we do. It is up to you and your care team to discern. You will have to make healthy and wise choices to survive and thrive with EDS. Most likely, you will need a team of support to help you manage your condition. Be open to help and be sure to get the help you need. We all need help sometimes. I did not do this alone.

For my child and every person with EDS that needs this.

May modern medicine give us answers and cures.
Until then, may ancient medicine sustain us.
And may we endure and live our lives to the fullest.

The 5 A's of Thriving With EDS Awareness

1. *Awareness,*
2. *Adjustments,*
3. *Acknowledgement,*
4. *Action,*
5. *and Acceptance*

*Bonus: Accommodations

WELCOME SURVIVORS AND THRIVERS!

"No one like you was ever born or ever will be."
—Constance Foster

Quandary: a state of perplexity or uncertainty over what to do in a difficult situation, a practical dilemma

Dear Reader,

If you are reading this book, most likely you or a loved one has been diagnosed with Ehlers-Danlos Syndrome (EDS). I am so glad that you have found this resource, which contains practical self-help techniques along with some motivational messages. I am not a medical doctor, so I cannot give specific medical advice. While I cannot counsel you or give you a program to follow to treat your unique situation, I can tell you what I learned along the way. I can also make you feel not so alone with EDS.

I found myself in a quandary with my EDS. And I had to find physicians, guides, videos, conferences, blogs, specialists, and other resources to help me navigate the struggles with a connective tissue disorder. If you have found yourself in a similar dilemma, this book will help you lessen your plight. Please take what resonates with you, take what is useful, and leave whatever doesn't fit your needs and unique situation. We have things in common but some of us have very different circumstances. You will have to balance out my wisdom with your own, based on your experiences of your type of EDS.

This book is designed to inspire you to thrive with EDS by first sharing my own story of survival. My hope is that you can keep going, live a great life, and know that you are not alone if you are suffering with this condition. On the other side of survival, there is true thriving with this condition. With this condition, you can go from surviving to thriving and back and forth. Like everything else in life, there are seasons and cycles of going through both experiences. As much as we strive for perfection, it is unreasonable to expect ourselves to be constant thrivers. Also, as you probably know, added pressure to overcome every health challenge and to be happy all the time is not good for us. It turns out that perfectionism is just added stress. So, I encourage you to remove any unreasonable expectations and self-inflicted stress. Having a positive mindset is helpful, but having a perfectionist mindset can be harmful.

I want my story to not only inspire you but also to provide emotional support for any fears with which you are struggling. Sometimes when we hear someone else's story, we can gather our own courage to face those fears and challenges. Even though connective tissue disorders have various presentations across demographics, we all share similar healthcare challenges—and headaches! The way we navigate those challenges can apply to universal experiences of the adversity we face. I noticed that there are common stages that we go through when confronted with a serious health issue.

I have designed this book according to the five major stages of my EDS recovery journey.

Here are my 5 A's to thriving/navigating EDS (plus a bonus):

1. *Awareness,*
2. *Adjustments,*
3. *Acknowledgement,*
4. *Action,*
5. *and Acceptance*
6. *Bonus: Accommodations

While I have numbered these A's, please know that I didn't apply these in order by any means. I simply noticed common underlying themes throughout my recovery journey with EDS and found some overlying steps of processing that were helpful to identify. I discovered that these were like stages at times. Interestingly, they were also very similar to the stages of grief processing. There are also the 3 A's of the 12 Step Recovery Programs that are very much the basis of my 5 A's. When I understood what I was going through, I felt more at peace with the process of healing my relationship with my EDS. I needed each one of these steps/stages to get me to the final step of appropriate **Action** with **Acceptance** while appreciating myself and continuing to make loving **Accommodations**. When I hadn't fully processed these steps, my actions were desperate, scattered, unfocused, and sometimes harmful. Also, you may notice that there is an action-oriented **A** after an emotional **A**. That's because we need to take action, even in small steps, to improve our changes and achieve better outcomes.

I encourage you to contemplate where you are with each of these five A's. You might currently be doing several good **Action** steps and yet still be stuck without answers. It happens. Just do the best you can and remember that your best may fluctuate.

On my EDS journey, I began to recognize the gaps in the medical system when it came to helping those with this condition. The medical community could almost diagnose EDS accurately, suggest physical therapy (for obvious reasons), and monitor and treat issues as they arose for me. However, there were many limitations that I observed. In my time, and in my area, I could not locate a connective tissue clinic or a physician that saw me as a whole person with uncommon problems and severe sensitivities. This meant that they were not thorough in creating my treatment plan because they didn't truly understand my rare condition's full cause or impact. My condition was very high-maintenance for me and for them. For that reason, rare and adverse things happened to me. I was lucky to have found a few amazing doctors on my path who helped me get to the next level of care. For them, I am forever grateful and consider them my heroes and angels sent from above.

As a yoga instructor for over ten years, I have also included **3 Starter Tips** (and some **Pro Tips**) to help you get started with helping yourself through your condition. Although yoga is considered a contraindication for people with EDS, I found that what the experts really meant was that stretching is not good for an already too flexible body. Stretching is not advised, and that needed to be made clearer to me. Plus, *over*stretching, just like *over*doing anything, is dangerous. Beyond stretching, my yoga practice consisted of strengthening poses, balancing postures, body awareness, proper physical alignment, meditation, and breathing techniques —these techniques allowed for relaxation, stress reduction, and much-needed sleep. My yoga practice sustained me for over twenty years with EDS and saved me when I was recovering from each health crisis. The year that I didn't do my type of safe yoga, my condition worsened.

Originally, when I read the top three contraindications for EDS (one of which was yoga) circulating online, I wanted to follow good sound expert advice, so I took a year off from practicing yoga. However, I deteriorated my physical, mental, emotional, and spiritual well-being with black-and-white thinking. As much as I wanted to follow the expert advice and improve my condition, I also had to follow my own guidance and what experience had taught me so far. Thus, I resumed a yoga practice that had a much gentler and more mindful focus for my EDS. I learned to adapt, modify, and completely refrain from many yoga postures and practices for safety reasons. Basically, I stopped doing headstands and showing off how flexible I was as a cool contortionist. I stopped turning my head almost completely around like an owl and purposefully limited any twisting movements. By being more mindful and restrictive, I was able to prevent bodily harm and injury and keep my practice going strong. I stopped trying to be like everyone else in the yoga world and stopped trying to keep up with other non-EDS teachers. It took a lot of self-acceptance to be able to stand firm in my beliefs. One thing that I believed in was yoga and its many health benefits.

After about a year, I saw how stopping my yoga practice decreased muscle tone and body awareness. It was simply too dangerous for me to quit being "in union" (a definition of yoga) with my body. The physical therapy that was prescribed was strenuous. I even sought out specialized EDS PT, and that required a six-hour, undoable drive. The best I could do was follow the book, ***Living Life to the Fullest with Ehlers-Danlos Syndrome: Guide to Living a Better Quality of Life***

While Having EDS by Kevin Muldowney, MSPT, and most importantly, my body's messages. This meant I had to step up my self-care and do things that supported me physically. I had to make many adjustments and personal modifications for exercises that were recommended. I ended up creating my own yoga practice for EDS, which I hope to offer in future videos on YouTube.

As I suffered and struggled with EDS, I began to understand the value of physical support and emotional support for any complex, chronic issue. This launched a heartfelt desire to serve others by writing this book. As I wrote, I felt like I was facing my painful past, complicated present, and uncertain future. I realized that all of my life was filled with such uncertainty, and I needed to find a way to survive and thrive within it. Outlining my story was a way to make peace with my past and give future generations my life experiences to draw from. My wish for you is that you take away at least one thing that makes your life with EDS better. Remember that you are uniquely designed, and there is no one else like you. That means you will have to tailor everything I write to fit your circumstances and situation. I may have several forms of EDS, so you may not identify with all my ailments or successes. So, please take what you can and leave the rest.

> *"It is not the strength of the body that counts,*
> *but the strength of the spirit."*
> —J.R.R. Tolkien

Sincerely,
Sonya Zappone
SonyaZappone.com

A BRIEF BUT LONG HISTORY

MY EDS JOURNEY TO —> DIAGNOSIS

Three Close Calls and Three Near-Death
*   Experiences*
"Nothing in life is to be feared, it is only to be
*   understood.*
Now is the time to understand more, so that we
*   may fear less."*
—Marie Curie, Polish-born scientist and the first
    woman awarded a Nobel Prize

A Puzzle With Many Pieces

I was a mystery for four decades. There were times when I was afraid, but each health catastrophe was a clue that something was seriously wrong. I knew something was odd when the most experienced doctors would tell me that an event (attributed to me) was rare. I watched them pace around the emergency room, looking very perplexed. I relied on those doctors for their expertise. I discovered it was a lofty expectation. I mistakenly thought doctors knew more than they actually did! I knew next to nothing medically when I began trying to piece it all together. My expectations led to many disappointments. I wanted my power back that I handed away to physicians. I wanted knowledge. I wanted to solve the mystery of myself, to put the puzzle pieces of me together, and be understood. I felt ashamed of complaining so much, of having so many incidents that landed me in the emergency room. So, I went on a mission for real answers. I was forty years old and already a survivor of many close calls and several near-death experiences. Marie Curie was right: "Now is the time to understand more, so that we may fear less."

Pro Tip:
   Learn as much as you can about yourself. Don't expect others to have all the answers.

Who Am I?

> "*Face your deficiencies and acknowledge them;*
>   *but do not let them master you.*
> *Let them teach you patience, sweetness, insight.*"
> —Helen Keller

I had so many different areas of my body affected that I had no idea how each piece fit into the puzzle of me. Every time something strange happened health-wise, I made a mental note of it. I was like a detective trying to solve a cold case that kept going. I was the unsolved mystery. I had no idea how all these strange physical maladies were related, but there was always one thing in common—me. They were all rare occurrences and were always bizarre. I was suffering physically, mentally, and emotionally. Sadly, most people were not compassionate. They were just as frustrated as I was, and some were downright dismissive. Others labeled me a hypochondriac, even if they didn't say it out loud or to my face. I never knew what I was going to get. Life was really a "box of chocolates." On the one hand, there were doctors and medical staff who were cold and insensitive to my plight, while on the other hand, I met doctors who I thought were saints or angels sent from above to save my life—a few times, just in the nick of time! I had to take the good with the bad. It was my only choice to stay alive. I had no idea what was going wrong with me. I felt helpless and had to rely on any doctor willing to help.

Invisible Illness

Things started to make sense for me when I was finally diagnosed at the age of thirty-nine with the connective tissue disorder Ehlers-Danlos Syndrome (EDS) - Hypermobility Type (hEDS). EDS is a rare collagen disorder that stems from genetic mutations, and while hypermobile is the most common subtype, it is also the least understood.

A geneticist made my diagnosis after a rheumatologist referred me to him in response to his suspicions. Once the geneticist saw how my arms, legs, and fingers easily bent backward, he asked if I would consider participating in some medical research (for which I eagerly donated my blood to science, wanting to find the biomarker). I pleaded with the geneticist to find the genetic marker as soon as possible because I had a seven-year-old daughter for whom I was concerned. I desperately wanted to know if I had unknowingly passed this condition on to her, but the truth was, I wasn't sure how much longer I would even be alive. I had so many brushes with death that I at least wanted to leave her with an answer for herself, not uncertainty. Did she inherit this from me? I prayed the answer would be a definitive "No." Leaving her with an answer was the least that I could do for her, and hopefully, this would help other EDS sufferers.

When my daughter showed me how her arms bent backward at the bus stop one day, my heart sank into the pit of my stomach. I, too, remember showing off my arms as a kid, not knowing what it meant. I was well aware, though, that getting her an accurate diagnosis could ultimately save her life. Even more so, it could save her sanity. I didn't want her to be treated like a hypochondriac and experience as many medical mishaps as I did. It felt like a hero's mission driving four and a half hours to the city for my genetics evaluation, seeking answers to my health dilemma. For my child, I would drive to the ends of the Earth. I investigated the limitations of scientific discovery the best that I could.

Revised Diagnosis

Two years before receiving my EDS diagnosis, a different genetics group diagnosed me with Generalized Joint Hypermobility Syndrome. I missed the EDS diagnosis by one question, which I ended up learning the answer to later that year. (Do you have any organ prolapse?) Plus, as more things started breaking down in my body, the longer I lived, the more boxes I could tick off on my medical checklist. Organ prolapse is a sad reality and happens with aging.

During my first visit to the geneticist, I had my blood drawn, and a connective tissue panel performed in the lab to identify my specific type of EDS. Unfortunately, at that time, a diagnosis for Hypermobility Spectrum Disorder (HSD) was only made possible by a process of elimination that ruled out all the other types. Currently, there are fourteen different subtypes and associated genes identified as the cause of EDS, and learning that I didn't have the others was a relief. I was very fearful of having vascular EDS (vEDS) since I was approaching forty. I was relieved to get the phone call from the genetics nurse letting me know that I didn't have that type. I remember taking a deep breath and sighing with relief. It was such an important moment that I remember exactly where I was standing. Vascular EDS shortens lifespans and is the most life-threatening.

The annoying problem with a diagnosis of the hypermobility type was that no gene had been identified yet. It was irritating that this could be the most common type of EDS, yet it had no identifiable biomarker. I was stuck with a debilitating disorder and in limbo between what science knew and had yet to discover, which meant that it was probably more complicated than a simple genetic "find." As I investigated, as I researched, I began to learn just how complicated health could be.

The good news was that my bloodwork showed two variants of connective tissue genes, ADAMTS2 and FLNA. These were essential clues for me; however, at the time, they were classified as "variants of uncertain significance," and as such, the geneticists couldn't tell me much, nor could they diagnose anything specific. The only advice I received from the first doctors was to participate in regular physical therapy for all my joint problems, which was not very helpful. It pointed me in the right direction because I would have to rely on my muscles, but it didn't give me a medication or supplement strategy, or any understanding of how or why my body was falling apart. I felt like I was flying blind, but at least I was still flying.

I was to follow up with the geneticists yearly and report on my condition. Finally, the genetics nurse *eventually* referred me to a more specialized geneticist after my numerous emails asking about recurrent infections that I experienced following my first abdominal surgery. I had so many questions because I needed to understand what was happening. When I asked her via email if I could have passed this on to my child, she said, "absolutely, you could have." It took me a year to reread her response because it was such a painful confirmation. I shuddered every time I thought of it, but blocking it out of my mind didn't make my EDS go away. I had to live on with this painful awareness. I needed courage to face the facts.

My second geneticist was a breath of fresh air. He wrote me a nine-page report on what to do and what to avoid. He was personally trying to find the HSD or hEDS biomarker in his lab. I was so glad to be able to contribute to science and meet someone who knew my disorder better than I did. Still, there was no cure for hEDS and no medication beyond pain meds. When I asked about my daughter, he explained that this was a dominantly passed gene meaning that all she had to do was inherit one bad copy of whatever gene caused this, and she would most likely be affected as well. Hearing that was heartbreaking for me. I suffered so much with this invisible condition—mentally, emotionally, physically, socially. I did not want this life for her.

Feeling Different

All my childhood, I knew that I was different. I was very bendy, prone to bruising, and was always sick with some type of infection that required antibiotics. I excelled in dance and gymnastics and was drawn to movement, but not to sports. I always seemed to become seriously hurt in any sport that I tried playing. I often rolled my ankles and had broken both of my feet over the years from falls. Accident-prone was my middle name. I learned to stay out of the way and be careful or risk getting hurt.

I never even attempted to be a waitress; I knew better. After all, I dropped, spilled, and accidentally broke things daily. Describing me as clumsy is an understatement.

My skin was also a constant daily dilemma. I picked at my scabs, which were prevalent across my body. My cuts always took a long time to heal and needed antibiotic ointment and bandages. I suffered from eczema and psoriasis, and my skin was covered in patchy dry spots that peeled and bled as a child. My father told me that I had "large pores like him" and to always rinse with cold water after a shower so they would close and not become infected or clogged. He was sort of right.

Boyfriends would comment on how I always had the softest skin of any girl they ever knew. Mothers at my yearly dance recitals would remark on my double-jointedness. I had no idea that these little things meant something big and would actually impact my health and life so severely later on. At the time, it was just cool to be different, unique, and noticed.

Always a Problem (Self-Esteem)

It seems like cruelty by design that I appear so normal on the surface, and yet underneath, I am not. Although people told me I was beautiful, I was plagued with acne. I always had scars and large, bloody, scary eruptions that made me ashamed of my skin. I had to work diligently to keep my face and body clear, though I often gave up and hid under hats and scarves or just stayed home. I would stop looking in the mirror because it was too painful to see what was happening from all my itching and picking. When I researched the ADAMTS2 gene, my skin issues finally made more sense. It was a skin-related gene. No wonder I was so soft and fragile! I was a slave to my skin issues, and the reason was my genetics! I didn't have to blame myself for not taking care of my skin, even though I always did because I was fighting an uphill battle. I was inherently different. Self-esteem obviously took a hit.

Pro Tip: Don't try to be "normal" like everyone else. Respect your limits.
<small>(Small print: at the same time, try to live a normal life and enjoy all you safely can)</small>

Before learning about ADAMTS2, the best I could do was hide under my clothing, even though clothes were another problem. I couldn't tolerate anything itchy, tight, or touching my skin, for that matter. I had to cut the tags off all my clothes. I could only wear soft, flexible things as I couldn't tolerate most fabrics. Shoes were a problem, as well. I could only wear certain types of shoes, or I would have more incidents of falling down or tripping. It was such a pain to shop for my body that I usually stayed with the same clothing and styles that worked for me, often ten years at a time. I always bought extra-large clothing, and even my family members picked on me for it. Many shopping sprees turned into failures, and I grew accustomed to the disappointment. However, when I found something that worked, I learned to stick with it. Some would say it was a blessing that I didn't love to shop because I have saved a lot of money, but I also didn't get to enjoy the pleasure of "retail therapy." Some curses can be blessings and vice versa!

What My Parents Told Me Growing Up

My parents were beyond clueless, even more than the doctors. All my parents told me was that I was always "itchy and gassy" as a kid, though they didn't know why. They said I had bad eczema. They noted how I was always on "the pink medicine" (antibiotics) and going to the doctor. They were often tired of my health issues and my complaining. I felt like a liability to them, not an asset. They also told me I was always getting hurt but never suspected anything aside from thinking I was just clumsy. They said I suffered from headaches, belly aches, and was in bed a lot. My pediatrician would see me often but only treated my ailments with courses of antibiotics and agreed with my parents that my injuries were due to my chronic clumsiness and typical childhood. Personally taking the blame for something that I couldn't help wore on my self-esteem. I suffered from self-doubt because what life was like for them (health-/wellness-wise) wasn't my personal experience. Discussions with my dad would leave me feeling incompetent. He would tell me that I was fragile and too sensitive. He often accused me of overreacting to things others thought were minor. Out of his frustration, he yelled at me to "toughen up" on a few occasions that required a strong, fit, able body. For me, little things were a big deal. Physical failure and my "incompetence" was my body talking, and no one was listening! When he suggested that I join the Airforce to pay for college, I laughed and asked him, "Do you really think I could survive bootcamp?" (There was just silence that followed.)

As you can guess, I missed many days of school due to illness. An ordinary cold would knock me down like the flu, and I always took longer to recover than my healthy friends. Despite this, though, I never really felt as if there was anything fundamentally wrong with me while growing up. I can look back and see how this affected my friendships. I was vulnerable and a target to those who tended to take advantage of others. But ignorance was bliss back then. In my teens, after years of dance, I gravitated towards yoga because it was super easy for me and made me feel good. I especially liked how slow it was and the resting time at the end of classes. It worked as a chosen form of exercise as well as a hobby for me.

First Jobs and Teenage Years

From the age of fourteen and a half, I worked many different jobs. Any job that required me to stand or sit for prolonged periods was too hard on my feet or back. I usually only lasted a year or two. I never knew why all this was a problem for me; I just knew that my body was high maintenance and I needed to move. I thought I was just "antsy" as people say... full of anxious energy so that I needed to fidget and move around regularly, so I naturally gravitated toward anything helpful to support my posture. I learned the value of wearing gel cushion insoles in my shoes to take the pressure off my feet and sleeping on memory foam mattresses to redistribute the weight of my body. I even found gel cushions for chairs. I tried anything that offered support for my body. I was also a fan of massage and loved them as much as I loved yoga. Yoga felt like an internal body massage to me, and it was how I coped with not having enough money to pay for regular massages.

By the age of sixteen, I suffered my very first health crisis, resulting in a week-long hospital stay where I was subjected to every test imaginable. The physicians, though, never discovered anything; they thought that I had a cyst on my ovary and was suffering from IBS and an allergic reaction to Bactrim. The results were "inconclusive"—a word that I came to hate and which left me with no way to help myself. That incident rendered me useless. I was sick for two months and missed so much school that my grades dropped from A's to C's. I barely passed the school year and was never able to regain my high grade point average. I could have been salutatorian (or close) if it wasn't for my illness that year. Thanks, EDS/MCAS mystery!

That episode was my first experience with medical mistakes and modern medicine's failure to detect the real issue. Going home from the hospital without answers was tough. My mom couldn't make sense of it either. She just chalked it up to me being allergic to onions; that's all she remembers from the ordeal. I remember the barium swallow and embarrassing colonoscopy. I remember the feeling of the pain medicine and how—for a few hours, at least—the extreme abdominal pain went away. It was wonderful to feel okay for a few hours. Going through that hospital visit and stay, I felt like there was something wrong with me; I just didn't know what that was. I cannot describe the feeling of being fundamentally flawed. It's emotionally painful and personally disappointing. I wanted to move on and forget that ever happened to me.

Yoga and a Holistic Approach

I began consciously adopting a holistic approach to my health and healing. It fit with the yogic teachings and lifestyle. I was drawn to yoga to relieve all the physical pain I tried to deny and suppress because others didn't seem to have the same experiences I did. I studied it intensely and became a certified yoga instructor. Becoming an instructor, though, wasn't my initial intention. I simply took the boot camp for my own personal health restoration. I figured that I could use it to help myself heal from a stressful desk job I took after college, when I noticed my health deteriorating. All I was doing was sitting at a desk, but it was rough on my body. It was not a good fit. Stress and sitting were my enemies.

The stretching component of yoga was the easy part for me; the hard part was the strengthening. I struggled to keep up with the cardio and endurance aspects in my yoga training but could impress everyone with my flexibility. During those yoga years, I had no idea why I was so flexible, but I felt like I fit in.

Even though I was trying to live a healthy lifestyle, I couldn't stop what happened to my body as I aged. At thirty-seven, I suffered a major health crisis, resulting in thirteen trips to the emergency room in fourteen days. My internal organs were in serious trouble, so I reluctantly had to rely on surgeons and modern medicine just to survive that year. If I count correctly, I needed twenty antibiotic prescriptions, three overnight stays for IV antibiotics, and two massive abdominal operations for my struggling internal organs. I opted to have five organs removed because we essentially didn't know what was happening to me. I wanted to stay alive, so I took extreme measures. The culprit was eventually located. A growth in my uterus attached to my c-section scar baffled everyone at the final hour.

After that ordeal, I then had to add my holistic approach back into my lifestyle and my new body. I had many years of training in vitamins from working at General Nutrition Center (GNC), which required learning about every vitamin on the store's shelves. I initially used that knowledge to stay thin in my twenties, but now I am using it as a means for survival. I honestly believe that learning all I did at GNC is how I made it this far, especially now that I see many younger women in their twenties with hEDS suffering so severely. I knew about protein intake and multivitamin benefits. I used the knowledge to live.

Pregnancy Problems

It wasn't until I was pregnant at age thirty-one that my health hit yet another critical turning point. To put it mildly, pregnancy hormones did not agree with my body in any way whatsoever. I was nauseous, bedridden, and bleeding for the entire gestation period. I even had to leave my job within the first two months due to severe morning sickness. At the time, though, we (me, my doctors, family) still didn't know I had EDS. Most people (doctors or family) assumed that I was just whining and complaining, which was even more cruelty I endured at the hands of healthy people.

I lost my vision during my last trimester because water filled both my retinas. Then, to add to my misfortune, during one of my exams, the nurse practitioner scraped my cervix, nearly sending me into preterm labor. I was bedridden in the hospital, moaning in pain and desperately trying to give my baby another four to six weeks in my womb, wanting to give her lungs a chance to develop. Staying alive was my first priority; the second was doing everything possible to carry my baby to full term, wanting so dearly to give her the best chance at life. I did whatever it took, no matter how harshly I was judged. My mom would bring me BLTs and apples—the two things my body and my baby craved. I surrendered to the needs of both of us.

My First "Close Call"/Traumatic Childbirth

Childbirth was a nightmare for me. Everything that could go wrong, did. I was just lucky that my baby and I didn't die, seeing how close we both came to it. I tried to put that behind me and never venture into the memory, or tears would fall for how much I missed out on what should have been a magical experience, not a near-death encounter. First of all, my water broke, but my contractions never began, and after testing positive for Group B Streptococcus (GBS), I ended up needing IV antibiotics just to give birth. After starting me on a course of antibiotics for the GBS, I was given Pitocin to start my contractions, making me feel like I was being sporadically electrocuted. I had tried to avoid this by waiting a day or two to see if things would happen naturally. I did all that I could to aim for a natural childbirthing experience. With that labor-inducing medication, my body would seize, and I would have contractions, though not uterine contractions, as I was supposed to have. It was pure modern-day medical torture and the reason I never had any other children. It ended up not dilating my uterus like it was intended to.

Another sign that things were unusual was that it took the top anesthesiologist three attempts to give me an epidural. This anesthesiologist was not just highly experienced, he was the one who trained others across the state. By the time he finally got the epidural in, it ended up just falling out. He told me that epidurals were usually not this difficult and that he didn't know why he was having so much trouble. I actually watched him scratch his head, perplexed and frustrated. I was losing faith in hospital medicine quickly.

After pushing for over five hours on my third day of labor, I was beyond exhausted and ultimately just surrendered to death as my eyes rolled back into my head, silently pleading for sweet relief. Pushing like our lives depended on it ruined my elbows, wrists, and knees. Once my doctors finally realized that I would not be able to deliver my baby vaginally, they finally ordered a cesarean section. Unfortunately, the anesthesia for the necessary cesarean section wore off immediately, leading me to scream at the doctors, desperate for them to stop cutting me open. My mother stood out in the hallway and listened in abject horror at my screams for mercy. I felt every cut the doctor was making. They finally realized that I needed full general anesthesia to complete the cesarean; thus, I never saw my baby girl being born. It is the number one heartbreak of my life.

After all of the trauma I went through to give birth, I ended up not making it out of the hospital for over a week afterward and experienced profuse postnatal bleeding. I also suffered immensely from a spinal fluid leak due to the numerous epidural attempts, resulting in a massive migraine. My recovery time was prolonged, and I was unable to hold or even see my baby for most of that time. Due to the strain of trying to push during vaginal delivery, my arms and hands were completely swollen and unusable, meaning that I couldn't be there for my new baby daughter. This was supposed to be the best time of my life, but it was honestly the worst. I could barely hold her to feed her from a tube. My breasts were cracked, bloody and raw, and so painful that I couldn't tolerate breastfeeding. I felt like a total failure but lucky to be alive. You could see the trauma in my eyes of my childbirth experience.

Perhaps even more traumatic than childbirth was that the doctors called Child Protective Services, saying that I couldn't take care of my baby due to my recovery. I couldn't, but that is not the point. They lacked understanding and mercy for a mother who just went through an incredibly traumatic childbirth and barely survived. They could have tried to help me find organizations who might have helped me care for my baby. Instead, my mother had to quit her job to care for my daughter and me. At least now I could finally take my daughter home. We had no idea that I had EDS. I believe this further traumatizing event would have never happened had they known I was struggling with a complex connective tissue disorder.

Looking back now, it's clear that they would have never put me through all of those days of labor with a heart condition and an underlying genetic disorder. Somehow—gratefully—we both survived, and I whispered to my baby when they placed her on my bare chest for skin-to-skin contact, "Life can only get better for us, from this point on." It was certainly true seeing just how much we went through.

Important Medical Decisions

I knew that my childbirth was a close call, and it made my decision not to have any more children much easier, even though it was emotionally difficult to admit my physical limitations. It was the right decision for my health, but changed the future that I thought I would have as a mother. I had to face my limitations once again.

Because I knew that I would not make it through another pregnancy and childbirth, I needed to decide how to avoid it. I had very bad side effects from birth control in the past. I could not tolerate taking hormones like progesterone or estrogen. I experimented with many other kinds of birth control, and all of them were too difficult to deal with. I decided to have a tubal ligation. When the surgeon told me he (or she) could remove my fallopian tubes entirely instead of using metal clips as was customary, I immediately agreed, knowing that metal and my body would be a bad combination. After all, my skin already had many issues with metal, so I had no reason to believe my internal organs would fare any better.

I remember the moment that I told my parents my decision not to have any more children. I had to let go of a dream to have a son, and I cried. They didn't understand such a drastic measure, but I knew all too well the risk of death I would be facing if I were ever to get pregnant again. I needed to live for my daughter. She was my future as I was hers, and she mattered more than any dream of another child.

Second Close Call

Unfortunately, childbirth wasn't my only brush with death. To help my body heal after the abuse of labor, I visited a chiropractor. However, during the routine neck adjustment, something went horribly wrong. I was suddenly severely dizzy and couldn't get up off the table. I had to be rushed by ambulance to the emergency room. It turns out that I suffered from a slight muscle tear. I was lucky that it wasn't a vertebral artery tear, which can cause a stroke or even death. It could have easily been that. Many doctors cringed when I told them I went to a chiropractor.

Again, I didn't know I had EDS at the time. I had no idea that pregnancy, chiropractic care, or yoga were contraindicated for my condition. I was "flying blind." It was another very close call. It took a while to digest and realize what almost happened to me. I iced my neck and waited for it to heal. I thanked my lucky stars for being alive and that my neck wasn't broken. I researched chiropractic injuries and found that this was a serious issue and a known risk with neck adjustments and chiropractors. It was incredibly risky and dangerous for someone with my condition, even if I didn't know about my EDS at the time. I was just desperate for natural remedies and for someone to fix me. I never considered taking control of my health decisions; I relied on professional advice and help.

Physical Therapy Injuries

After childbirth, my bladder leaked, so I was prescribed physical therapy, unaware that it would aggravate my as-of-yet undiagnosed EDS. I had a great therapist who worked me hard with many lower body exercises. I always walked away sweaty and complained to her that it seemed as if I had to work out harder than all of the other people in the therapy room. After a few months, I mentioned that kneeling was too hard on my knees, so we had to stop those particular exercises. Then one day, while I was attempting a lunge with a small weight, I heard my left knee pop! I had no idea what happened, but I had to take months off from my therapy. I discovered that I had dislocated my knee, which even today chronically slips out of joint. I learned the hard way that I could never overextend a lunge, nor add any additional weight to my joints. If we had known that I had EDS, we would have designed a more gentle regimen.

Gym Injuries

Because I felt so floppy, I used weight machines to try to strengthen my body. I joined a gym and hired a personal trainer. One day while pushing myself too hard without the supervision of my trainer, I heard another pop, this time in the middle of my back. I was trying to lift seventy pounds while twisting myself to handle the extra weight. In doing so, I snapped a ligament in my spine. However, when I went to the emergency room, they took an x-ray of the wrong part of my back, and I was ultimately sent home with only muscle relaxers.

To this day, the middle of my spine (the exact location) remains a point of instability, and I struggle to lie down at night as the bones in my back will pop and slide from side to side. I also stopped being able to lie on my left side because my spine would slip, causing me to wake up with my heart racing as I gasped for air. I was beginning to learn that every injury I sustained would end up haunting me for the rest of my life. I had no idea why these minor issues would not heal fully or properly.

Due to this injury, and still not knowing about my elusive EDS diagnosis, I learned that I could not train with heavy or moderate weights. I realized that I should not attempt to push my body beyond its physical limitations, or else any injury that I might receive would never truly heal. It was a new reality that I was facing, and it was awful to think about.

Near-Death Experiences: *Urinary Tract Infection (UTI), Gallbladder Malfunction, Pelvic Inflammatory Disease, or All Three?*

At thirty-seven years old, I had a major health crisis that still haunts me to this day. Fearing that I was dying, I drove myself to the emergency room thirteen times in thirteen days. I had severe upper and lower abdominal pain. No one understood why and doctors couldn't find a cause. I would point to the localized areas of my pain, but every CT scan I had did not reveal the source of pain.

Finally, I was given antibiotics which seemed to help for a week, but then I would become sick once again. I couldn't eat or sleep and was tirelessly searching for doctors who could give me answers. I went to the hospital so often that I ended up being admitted three times to receive IV antibiotics, which only helped for a while before I would get ill all over again. I felt like I was clinging on to life, and no one knew why. It was baffling. I was in reaction mode and hyper-alert. I felt like I was struggling to take each breath. I could not relax, and it felt like life or death daily.

Finally, I drove to an out-of-state hospital that admitted me. Once there, an experienced surgeon examined me with an ultrasound and found that the wall of my gallbladder was thickened. This reminded me of a memorable gallbladder attack after consuming Chinese food containing MSG the previous year. I had stopped eating that food and switched to more salads but didn't pursue more testing. I wanted to try to heal myself with an all-natural diet.

Aside from my gallbladder issue, they found a large cyst on one of my ovaries. In a desperate attempt to save my life and stop whatever was happening, I had both the ovary and gallbladder removed, along with my appendix. It was an extreme situation, but I had already been hospitalized three times to receive double IV antibiotics as I begged for life. I was living from morphine injection to morphine injection just to withstand both the lower abdominal pain and this sickening feeling that I could only describe as some sort of "intolerable illness" throughout my body. When my gallbladder was removed, it showed a rare disease of non-pigmented stones, so I thought that must have been the cause. I still didn't know that I had EDS.

After having those three organs removed, I was only healthy for one month before getting sick yet again. I assumed it was a urinary tract infection (UTI) since I had so much diarrhea from the gallbladder removal as my liver struggled to regain balance and control of the digestive process. It was a common side effect of not having the gallbladder to regulate liver enzymes and salts. I went from doctor to doctor and gynecologist to gynecologist, but they seemed just to consider me crazy, and I certainly felt like I was. I was sick, and no one could find a cause until a urologist finally took a look inside me with a tiny camera and saw a bulging growth from my uterus that was protruding into my bladder.

I was then sent back to a gynecologist because it wasn't a recurring UTI, as previously thought. I needed another massive abdominal surgery —an emergency hysterectomy. The weirdly confusing thing was that it appeared as if my C-Section scar ruptured and had grown what looked like some sort of cord with a suspicious growth hanging on the end, which was embedded in my uterus. On top of this, I already had adeno-myosis, which was a thickening of my uterine wall. I desperately tried to hang on for dear life and was put on antibiotics until I could be sched-uled for my surgery.

I felt so overlooked by my doctors that I ended up going to a different OB/GYN rather than return to any of the previous nine who missed the diagnosis and ultimately dismissed my health concerns. I opted for the most experienced physician available: the head of the department himself. After the urologist that I trusted found a large cyst on my other ovary, I requested that my new OB/GYN remove it for me as well. Despite already deciding not to have any more children, this operation was just another massive loss for me.

The post-op recovery was one of the most challenging things that I had to go through in my life. I was laid out in bed for months on end, trying to heal my stitches to the point where they wouldn't break open. After eight grueling months, I still had unhealed stitches and granulation tissue. This told me that I was healing extremely slowly. I ended up requiring several rounds of antibiotics for the infections I unfortunately developed during the healing process.

In case it was hard to tell, my thirty-seventh year was an absolute blur, and I kept thinking that I was lucky to have lived. Two abdominal surgeries and six organ removals later, I was alive and thankful to be a mother. I still had a young child to raise who needed me, so I fought to stay alive for her even when I felt like giving up and succumbing to death many times, both at home and in the ER and hospital.

I was so tired of running to the emergency room, telling the doctors that I felt like I was dying only for them to send me away with Tylenol, probably because they suspected that I was just seeking drugs. I felt like I was near death or dying for so many months that I was completely traumatized. I was continually driving to different hospitals, trying to get a second opinion. I had six x-rays in two months. It was a herculean effort and an insane year. If it wasn't for my persistence, I would have died, not knowing that I had EDS.

So Many Questions

When I added together all these bizarre health and medical mysteries, I began to wonder what was wrong with me. I realized that I just had a health crisis like none I had ever seen in my family. I was sent to every doctor for every test until I finally went to a rheumatologist who noticed I had a rare condition called Ehlers-Danlos Syndrome. It was finally an answer. It confirmed that something was underlying these events.

How Did He Figure It Out? What Did He Do Differently?

He took the time to listen and not judge me. His brilliance sent me to genetic specialists, where I was finally given the sanity-saving diagnosis. I owe my life to this rheumatologist. But now I had so much medical trauma to recover from that living another day didn't feel guaranteed anymore. I began a medical journey that I never thought I would have to take while being so "young." Life changed dramatically.

After my EDS diagnosis, I was more mindful, but I still didn't fully understand my condition. I was more restrictive in my daily activities but was determined to live a normal life. That was until my second neck injury, when my life changed drastically. This health crisis was even more severe than the year of my two abdominal surgeries, numerous ER trips, and multiple hospitalizations for IV antibiotics. It was a game-changer.

Third Close Call

I was just starting to get back to living my life when I went on a retreat and slept in a bunk bed with the wrong pillow. I woke up with extreme neck pain. In an attempt to stretch, I turned my head hard and felt something snap off in my neck. I was suddenly so dizzy that I couldn't get up. I needed help. My parents had to come to get me as I couldn't drive. I ended up having to cancel the rest of my expensive relaxing weekend. I cried to my roommates that I didn't know what was happening.

Once I was back home, I went to the ER and underwent various scans and imaging. Fortunately for me, I didn't tear a vertebral artery or have any other identifiable radiological findings. However, every time I laid back at night or tipped my head backward, my vision would fade, and I would feel like I was losing consciousness. This time the emergency doctor took me seriously with a confirmed diagnosis of EDS, though they still never found anything in the imaging to report. I was so restricted with neck movements that it consumed my entire night and day trying to avoid the positions that caused the neurological issues.

Trying to find an answer, I searched all over New England for neurosurgeons and EDS specialists for a year. I finally discovered that I had a common condition/comorbidity called Cranio-Cervical Instability (CCI) due to my hEDS. Unfortunately, the only remedy is a fusion surgery, called Cranio-Cervical Fusion, and I would have to wear a hard neck brace indefinitely. Learning that this was a common unfortunate co-occurrence really depressed me.

I Wanted to Know Why

As time went on, and as I lost the ability to hold my head in place due to ligament failure, I knew I needed the most horrific-looking fusion to stabilize my skull to my cervical vertebrae. I was so upset that I tried to blame myself, my EDS, and even the tiny bit of estrogen HRT supplement I was taking for my hysterectomy to avoid menopause, but the blame didn't matter. Blame and fault-finding wouldn't glue my skull to my cervical vertebrae to keep my head from falling off or slipping, pinching off nerves, or possibly severing the carotid or vertebral arteries running to my brain. I was now permanently disabled and was not confident that I could survive another major surgery at age forty.

I researched this neurosurgery night and day and found that women with hEDS who commonly needed this procedure had indeed died from it. To add insult to injury, I had to face the reality that the two top neurosurgeons performing this procedure in the US weren't covered by my health insurance. It was a $250,000 procedure that often resulted in needing even more fusions down the spine due to Adjacent Segment Disease (ASD). My options were limited and extremely expensive, both financially and physically. Corrective surgery was far-fetched and out of reach.

Due to my previous physical therapy and gym injuries that never fully healed and still plagued me, I suspected that my cervical ligaments would probably pose a similar problem for me. Facing my new reality, I lost hope of living my normal life. My injuries were piling up, and I was getting older. EDS was here to stay, and I couldn't ignore my diagnosis any longer.

I officially knew that I had EDS.

> *"Self-preservation is the first principle of our nature."*
> —Alexander Hamilton

Living with Cranio-Cervical Instability (CCI)

My new health problems were real, scary and severe. My life had to change. I was now disabled from that second neck injury and hEDS. Life was suddenly very different and very restrictive. I needed a hard neck brace, a wheelchair for my dizzy days, and ski poles to aid my walking whenever I was able to do so. I was unable to work due to the headaches, fatigue, and debilitating dizziness that plagued me. I could no longer count on my body to hold itself together, so I learned to wear braces for every joint and stopped bending over.

I began physical therapy targeted specifically for those with EDS. My new physical therapist had to learn how to help me while I learned how to help myself. He couldn't manipulate my head or neck, which some people said would help, but I instinctively knew it would be dangerous. He respected the condition and understood the fine line of fragility that I walked daily. I did what I could, knowing very little but at least knowing something.

Looking back, I now find it appalling that doctors first thought I had inner ear crystals and wanted me to do neck and head range of motion exercises and prescribed antibiotics for a possible inner ear infection. Although that would be a more common cause of dizziness, I knew now that I had EDS. All they had to do was look the condition up online like I did, and they would see this comorbidity as a huge risk factor. I would have been spared the ruling-out process and years of uncertainty.

A Mast Cell Activation Disorder/Syndrome (MCAD/MCAS) Connection

At age forty, I realized that my allergy condition was somehow linked to my joint instability. I discovered my MCAS and worked with an allergist. My MCAS was an untamed beast. It was bigger than all the other ailments I had, which included the cardiologist's findings of Grade II Diastolic Dysfunction and the association of Postural Orthostatic Tachycardia Syndrome (POTS) low blood pressure. None of those affected me as much as the MCAS. To tame the beast, I learned to avoid, avoid, avoid. I had extensive allergy testing, which showed I was allergic to milk, eggs, and wheat. It was like I wasn't allergic to anything but reacted to most everything. This was a strange beast, MCAS. Again, I had to go from doctor to doctor, seeking out answers until paying for comprehensive testing online to find the cause of my "allergy issues." I learned to pay for the answers that I needed. I found some answers that at least helped me be able to eat and avoid a feeding tube.

I was disappointed in the medical process of diagnosing maladies and injuries. The process was too lengthy and not nearly comprehensive enough. Doctors narrowly focused on one issue at a time and always started with the most common culprit, never considering more rare conditions. I knew I had EDS, but doctors still followed that old medical proverb by Theodore Woodward, professor at the University of Maryland School of Medicine: *"When you hear hoofbeats behind you, don't expect to see a zebra."* Using this method, I suffered greatly. I *was* a zebra that they didn't even screen for.

> *"In all things it is better to hope than to despair."*
> —Johann Wolfgang von Goethe

No Cure, No Treatment

There is still no cure for my hEDS. The only treatment suggested was muscle strengthening with PT to help stabilize my joints. Experts didn't know what caused it entirely, so they were not able to offer much else. So, I waited for massive neurosurgery, which no one, including myself, thought that I should undergo. Meanwhile, I met other women with all the same problems. Some had already experienced the surgery domino effect and were being held together with titanium. Others were waiting for better options. Some were trying the new technology of stem cell injections. I could see how desperate we all were based on how much we were willing to try.

Waiting for Neurosurgery or Something to Glue/Screw Me Together

COVID-19 made me face my mortality yet again. I didn't know if I would survive an exposure. Looking even further down the road, I don't know if I will survive the Cranio-Cervical Fusion surgery if I decide to do it. So, I decided to write this book in hopes that I could help others. I made it my mission to share my wisdom, insight, and encouragement with other EDS survivors. I also don't know if my daughter inherited this and will need my insight and experience when she is older. I want to pass on every helpful life-saving tip and strategy to her and others. Mostly, I want to leave something loving for her, and apologize for not realizing that I would be leaving her with something like this. At the very least, I want to warn her. At best, I want to educate her and give her an essential guide.

> *"You gotta be your own detective sometimes.*
> *Geesh!"*
> —a journal entry

I am still on a mission to get a full picture of my health, no matter how complicated. I need answers to live as long as I can for my daughter. I want to be as healthy and as drug-free as possible. I know the keys to my health issues are 1.) genetics and 2.) chemical reactions. By trial and error, I learned that everything is a chemical reaction to be taken seriously and given thought —every choice matters, including sleep, relaxation, and rest. Food and supplements are significant factors too. I am wise enough to know that drugs are only for temporary relief and not to be relied upon, if at all possible. I came to this personal conclusion after suffering so many serious side effects from drugs. One thing always led to another. I have to be mindful of what medication I take, how much and how often. Everything needs considerable mindful deliberation. Each choice matters.

An EDS Survivor Story

It is clear to me that I have narrowly survived EDS. I have suffered severe medical trauma, and thought it would be important for others to hear my story. People say that strength is built through hardship, so I must be strong. However, I know COVID-19 is lurking, and I have Blood Type A with several underlying health conditions. I know that going forward, I have to be my own detective. I also have to be a pioneer for other EDS women. I felt this overwhelming and urgent need to tell my story and share my experience, strength, and hope with whoever needs it. Time is ticking. This is the push that made me want to share my wisdom. I hope my story emotionally supports you as you write your own.

> *"That which does not kill us makes us stronger."*
> —Friedrich Nietzsche

KEY #1

AWARENESS

"I choose not to place 'DIS' in my ability."
—Robert M. Hensel

FIRST THINGS FIRST
BE AWARE AND BEWARE!

AWARENESS

Becoming aware of Ehlers–Danlos Syndrome [EDS] is the first step towards accepting the diagnosis, which leads to true/proper adjustments and then clear/proper action.

(The 5 A's: Awareness, Acknowledgement, Adjustments/Action, and Acceptance)

> *"Consequences are governed by principles, and*
> *behavior is governed by values,*
> *therefore, value principles!"*
> —Stephen R. Covey, *First Things First*

The Ultimate Goal Is Acceptance, but First Comes Awareness

I had a very hard time accepting my EDS diagnosis, even after the genetic confirmation with undeniable blood work indicating the presence of two connective tissue-type mutations. I thought I wouldn't struggle with this part because it validated so many excruciating experiences that came with living in my EDS body. None of that mattered to me emotionally, though. Emotionally, it was hard to accept the EDS diagnosis. I denied it for a few years and kept it a secret from everyone. I didn't even take the diagnosis out of my mind to look at it and filed away the paperwork hoping that somehow it would go away. I was aware but not fully aware of what hEDS meant. I experienced some type of shock and couldn't reframe my life and future based on this new knowledge.

To cope, I practiced denial so my diagnosis never really sunk in. I learned that denial was a short-term coping mechanism employed to help me deal with overwhelming information, but in reality, it is a terrible long-term strategy for survival. I started to rely on the wisdom of Stephen Covey, author of *First Things First* and began applying this principle to dealing with my condition and situation as I lived on with EDS.

> *"We are free to choose our actions, . . . but we are*
> *not free to choose the consequences of these*
> *actions."*
> —Stephen R. Covey, *First Things First*

Denial worked (somewhat) until my second serious neck injury. Denial kept me living life rather than shriveling up into a state of fear and depression. But as I learned the "hard way" . . . denial can be deadly. If mission control was my brain, then I was running the risk of losing everything with these neck injuries. I risked losing control of my body, vision, hearing, and thought-processing due to injury to the arteries feeding my brain's blood supply. It was one thing to break my foot from my ankle rolling over (which happened often). It would be quite another to break my neck and be so dizzy that I couldn't drive or lay my head back at night to sleep, or worse, tear an artery to my brain and be found dead!

I found my "rock bottom" with the second neck injury. I was, for the most part, incapacitated by it. I was homebound and helpless in a lot of ways. I had the fear and risk of further injury hanging over my head—quite literally. It took many months to begin recovery and, in some areas, up to a full year to heal a torn ligament or tendon. I stopped trying to figure out what kept snapping when an injury occurred. I was getting so much radiation from x-rays that I decided to just live with most of the injuries and let my primary doctor know about them the next time something landed me in her office.

The neck injury took precedence over any sprain to any other joint. It was just so darn serious. It stopped me from living my life for a full year as I went on a mission to find a surgeon who could screw my head onto my neck.

> *"What we believe about ourselves and our*
> *purpose has a powerful impact on how we*
> *live, how we love, and what we learn."*
> — Stephen R. Covey, *First Things First*

No Cure / Limited Treatment = Chronic Illness

I met a pain doctor who was one of the most practical doctors that I had ever met. Through working with him, I finally got the message that I had a chronic illness and that, unfortunately, I wasn't just gifted with fabulous flexibility. I liked how much he thought about my treatment for EDS all the way through. Many options I wanted to try for temporary relief had the potential to create long-term problems for me. After traveling from doctor to doctor, it became clear that there was no easy solution to living with EDS. More importantly, there was no cure. Even though I endured an unacceptable amount of pain, doctors sent me home with nothing that could help me other than a few words. I appreciated him because he knew more about connective tissue disorders than any doctor I had ever met in my area. I appreciated that he didn't just think in terms of knees and elbows but all the connective tissue of my body.

When he used the words "chronic condition" and "life-long," it really hit me. I cried all the way home from the appointment, realizing he was right. EDS was not going away. I had finally become fully aware. The only thing he could offer was a strong suggestion to do physical therapy and stick with it like my life depended on it because, quite frankly, it did. My muscles mattered.

"Best way to predict your future is to create it."
—Stephen R. Covey, *First Things First*

Second Pain Doctor Appointment

During a follow-up session, my doctor repeated the physical therapist's name he had mentioned in a prior visit. I realized I had "dropped the ball" and never followed up by doing PT like he said the first time. He and I agreed that pain medication wouldn't solve my problem structurally. We agreed that Tylenol and natural remedies were my first line of defense and needed to be my first choice because of my stomach sensitivities (lining tears from weak collagen) as well as to prevent unwanted side-effects (from Mast Cell Activation Syndrome [MCAS]) reactions.

I needed his guidance and rational thought because I was just too emotional. He spoke to me with logic, common sense, and reason at a time when I was extremely confused and caught up in my grief over the prognosis. I was swirling with emotions that I had never felt before. It was a mixture of despair, hopelessness, fear, anxiety, heartache, heartbreak, grief, relief, and a tiny bit of hope. I didn't have a name for this complex feeling. I felt like I just received the news that I had abruptly turned ninety years old and my life would be cut short. And if my life was not cut short, I would certainly suffer in pain with many, many problems. The tiny bit of hope was there because I finally had a diagnosis and wouldn't be called "crazy" anymore. I appreciated that more than anyone could ever understand– unless you have EDS yourself and suffer a multitude of problems where people get sick of hearing you complain.

I saw him that second time to ask him if he would help me if I got the CranioCervical Fusion operation for my craniocervical instability. I would need his help if I ended up in more pain than I could handle. I was worried about facing excruciating pain that couldn't be solved by popping things back into place. How could I deal with the pain if I couldn't pop my neck bones back into place manually, and I was fixed/screwed into position? He looked at me straight in my eyes, which were filled with horror and tears, and said, "You don't want that baggage from a fusion." Deep down, I knew he was right, but I had a sense of urgency and desperation in my bones to fix them in place or die. I allowed his words to haunt me.

> *"What you alone can contribute, no one else can*
> *contribute. Viktor Frankl said we don't*
> *invent our mission; we detect it. It's within us*
> *waiting to be realized."*
> —Stephen R. Covey, *First Things First*

On the way home, I realized I needed emotional support to help me deal with my EDS. This was hard to handle. It was tough to face all of my raging and ranging emotions. I was facing a life sentence of health issues and painful injuries. I was facing major restrictions on all my activities. I was facing a different life than I planned or wanted for myself. I was facing the rapid deterioration of my body. I had to accept and adjust while grieving the loss of my life that I was living pre-diagnosis, pre-second neck injury.

I needed support on my journey to a healthy level of acceptance. I also needed to stop blaming physical therapy for my previous knee injury, which occurred during a session, and find the motivation to resume participation in the new/revised/much gentler recommended PT programs. I had hurt myself doing moves that were too hard on my joints; now I knew why. I tried to stop blaming myself with daily self-talk that the previous therapy had happened before I knew I had EDS. Going forward, I would be more careful and more aware. PT wasn't the problem; doing too much and being too hard on my body was.

> *"Doing more things faster is no substitute for*
> *doing the right things."*
> — Stephen R. Covey, *First Things First*

New Hope

The next morning, an epiphany came during my morning meditation. I started with an inspirational reading that talked about a simple yet profound parable that Jesus told. It was the one about building a house on sand or stone. Although not religious, I often attended churches hoping to hear a message that would help me survive EDS and hang on. It was a simple story reminding us that the rain and winds of life come to everyone's house at some point. However, those built on stone will still be standing when the storm ends.

I found some similarities to my situation. I needed to be still standing because I had a young child to raise who still needed me. I needed to make my body my "bedrock." Physical therapy could help get me there. Being practical and taking advice could also help get me there. I knew that life was going to happen; the rains would fall, the winds would blow. I needed to build my house to be strong if I was going to have a chance of standing. I could thrive with EDS if I listened to my body and to this one practical doctor's wisdom. I began walking every day, and I started physical therapy with my new diagnosis dictating my limits. I searched for a specific PT program for EDS and found one. I had new hope.

Once full awareness of my condition kicked in, my self-guiding principles for thriving with EDS became:

- Do, but don't overdo.
- Accept my limitations and always work around them.

> *"It's not enough to dream. It's not enough to try.*
> *It's not enough to set goals or climb ladders.*
> *It's not enough to value. The effort has to be*
> *based on practical realities that produce the*
> *result. Only then can we dream, set goals,*
> *and work to achieve them with confidence."*
> —Stephen R. Covey, *First Things First*

Self-Coaching Suggestions:

1. What would fully accepting your diagnosis mean for you?
2. What do you have to reconsider in your life that doesn't fit with your current diagnosis?
3. What is most important for your health and well-being?

*"The struggle comes when we sense a gap
between the clock and the compass—when
what we do doesn't contribute to what is
most important in our lives."*
—Stephen R. Covey, *First Things First*

AWARENESS 101

PROTECTED BY KNOWLEDGE

DO: Increase your Awareness.

Increasing my awareness of my condition and comorbidities protected me from further harm. The knowledge of contraindications and the potential catastrophes of certain surgeries helped keep me safe at the medical level. Knowing things that were relevant to EDS or MCAS was super important. Turning away from EDS and not staying informed and "in the know" was so dangerous. I repeat: denial is dangerous. I heavily researched my condition when I realized that there was much more to me than I realized. There was so much to learn and become aware of, things that I never even fathomed. But then, who can fathom someone's head sliding off and bones falling out of sockets randomly anyways?

DO: Learn the art of EDS survival from others.

Life is very much about survival and mostly survival of the "fittest." Well, what happens when you're not one of the "fittest," physically speaking? What can you do to ensure your survival among those hearty, solid, stable folk? You can educate yourself, seek out information, learn, and become aware. I did this by doing my own internet search and reading many books to see what approaches fit for me and my type of EDS case.

Within a year, I ended up knowing more about my condition than most physicians. I had watched the lives of other EDSers on YouTube and saw firsthand what I was dealing with. It was a crash course in the pitfalls of EDS. It was very validating because I found it genuinely interesting and because this topic hit home. This information was about something that I lived with for years, something I was born with. I came across mostly young girls with the EDS/MCAS combo, detailing their lives of medical intervention after medical intervention... all desperately seeking answers, solutions, and permanent fixes. I felt their agony and struggle. I had gone through most of it, and what I hadn't, they were doing ahead of me. It was like watching a medical experiment firsthand and seeing the outcomes. Sure, we all live with a level of uncertainty, but there are ways to live with more clear vision.

DON'T: Hurt yourself by being ignorant and uninformed.

Burying my head in the sand wasn't helpful. Not facing EDS and being able to see what I was up against limited my knowledge. When we go through something blind, we tend to hit many walls, but when we research and read up on the issues, we walk with clear and conscious vision.

I found it extremely important to understand the diagnosis —not just the name, but the cause or causes and the implications. Finding the root cause can be the "game-changer" when it comes to medical treatment. Instead of shutting up a struggling system (the body), you can assist it in healing. For example, if you discover that gluten leads to inflammation, and that inflammation affects your joints more severely, you have the knowledge to change this. Further, if you discover you lack a gene (MTHR) to properly methylate B vitamins and detox your body, you can take the right type of vitamins to balance this out. Or, if you find out that you are allergic to sulfa drugs, then you can avoid them. Putting steroids, painkillers, and other stopping drugs onto a burning fire provides only temporary relief. It's not a permanent fix.

There is so much power in knowledge. The power to self-protect being the main one. There is also power in putting your knowledge into play. By living with wisdom, you can avoid further harm and seek out correct treatments. If the doctors don't know, you don't have to accept hopelessness. You can search and seek out someone who does, or even better, look for that knowledge yourself.

DO: Take time to research your health-related matters.

This may seem very basic or obvious to you, but there are those out there who rely entirely on doctors' advice and limited knowledge. Rare conditions call for a more proactive and protective approach. There aren't many experts, and it gets very complicated when comorbidities pile atop more comorbidities. Even more so, as we age, we have to contend with not just the odd health crisis, but the normal health issues that happen to even the typical person. So take the time to do this type of studying and think of it as continuing education. Do it for yourself and your future. Do it because you matter and are worth it. Yes, there may be a lot more questions than answers as you start, but the longer you live (with awareness), the better you can be at solving some of these mysteries yourself—especially when it comes to food and medications. Trial-and-error methods have helped scientists and people for thousands of years. These personal experiments are not only educational but provide a foundation. If someone has personally explored EDS/MCAS or whatever variation you suffer, they most likely presented this information to the world so that others can learn. Make room in your life for lifelong research and findings. It can be a lifesaver.

DO: All you can to protect your health!

(Even if this means you become almost like an in-resident doctor yourself!)

> *"So you're a little weird? Work it! A little*
> *different? OWN it.*
> *Better to be a nerd than one of the herd."*
> —Mandy Hale

MAKING ADJUSTMENTS WITH AWARENESS

THRIVING WITH EDS

3 Starter Tips
(Listen, Be Aware, Stay Mindful)

Thriving sounds so much better than surviving, right? Before I jump into all my survival strategies, here are some of my helpful tips and suggestions for thriving with EDS. Please take what you like and leave the rest. Some of this may be just what you need at the moment.

Tip #1: Listen to Your Body

To thrive with Ehlers–Danlos Syndrome, I learned to listen to my body's messages. Ignoring my body led to many unnecessary injuries, dislocations, strains, tears, handicaps, and permanent physical problems that might have been otherwise avoided. After learning this valuable lesson the hard way, I decided to adopt a new mantra: "I listen to my body. I listen to my body. I honor and listen to my body, damn it!"

So no matter what others may have suggested as solutions for me, it always came down to my own inner wisdom and trusting my gut. My body always had the final say, anyway. If my body couldn't do something, it just simply couldn't do it. You can't use a drill sergeant approach when your body is jelly! No one could argue with the truth. To avoid the consequences of not listening to my body, I learned to <u>listen</u>—intently— as well as honor any pain messages. So, I encourage you to start listening to yours. Your body has innate survival intelligence. Once you learn to listen, then you have to honor what you hear. Hearing something and rushing to the medicine cabinet is the same thing as telling the body to "shut up!" So, be kind, be gentle, and have some self-compassion. (FYI: most likely, you will hear the pain.)

Important Lesson #1: Pain is a Message!

Tip #2: Increase your Awareness / Notice What Hurts

This can seem counterintuitive, but pain is my friend. I learned to appreciate pain as a messenger. It turned out that pain was not my enemy my whole life; it was my friend with a message. I learned to thank my pain for telling me that something was amiss rather than get mad about having pain. Fearing and loathing my pain just kept me anxious and running from my own body. I would rush to the medicine cabinet for pain meds, not realizing that the pain was a flag, a warning, a sign. Now, when I feel pain, I lovingly listen and investigate before managing it. I use a strategy of starting with non-medication options to avoid more side-effect problems. So, I start with positional therapy, physical movements, heat, and naps. I have even distracted myself from pain by watching movies to see if it is something that will pass. The body can amazingly heal/fix itself. Sometimes I just needed to give it the time in which to do that.

I am amazed at how impatient we are with the human body. Everything in society tells us that a quick fix is the best way to keep us functioning. But that "more, free, fast and now" approach isn't in line with our nature. Sometimes a real "time-out" from life to convalesce and heal is the true remedy.

> **Con·va·lesce:** to recover one's health and strength over a period of time after an illness or operation or anything traumatic

Listening With Love

Self-compassion really is the solution to our suffering. So, I encourage you to listen with love to the pain, learn to sit with it, before medicating it immediately to "shut it up." What is it trying to tell you? Is there a joint out of place? Are you weak in the legs and need to adopt a strengthening program? Have you not moved in a few days, and have things started to compress and pinch nerves or discs? Where is the pain originally coming from? Don't be shy about asking your body questions. It is important to know what it is trying to tell you.

I always remember that pain is a signal making me aware of something happening in the body. I even learned that it could indicate healing after surgery and it doesn't always mean something awful has happened. So, try to get as many specifics as you can. Go for the details. Sometimes the answers and solutions come from the little things. Honor the message of pain where you can and build it up into a healthy habit of identifying signals from yourself. Try to increase your awareness by diving into what the pain is saying versus trying to avoid it. With awareness, you can take appropriate action or make adjustments, even if the action is resting and doing nothing—that is still an appropriate action sometimes.

Avoiding pain with EDS can be dangerous and, quite frankly, not possible. This doesn't just apply to EDSers, it's true for every human body—just more so for us and others like us. So, make peace with pain and gain awareness to practice self-preservation, self-protection, and self-partnering.

(Basically, get really good at noticing things. Then, you will get good at connecting the dots and finding out the problems.)

Tip #3: Practice Mindfulness and Injury Prevention

With EDS, you will have to be mindful of your movements to avoid injuring yourself. Mindfulness can extend to eating, activities, people, chosen careers, and every other choice in life. If you are mindful of when you need to rest, move/exercise, and avoid certain foods, then you can care for yourself in a better way and suffer less. Perhaps you could begin a food log. You could be mindful of how you position yourself in the shower and if you tip your head back too far. You could be mindful of your posture when sitting and if you slump and slouch while you drive. You could begin to be mindful if you are trying to do too much. You could extend mindfulness into every area of your life to bring awareness to what you are doing as a habit, inadvertently, or subconsciously.

The dangers of not being mindful are too great to ignore. For example, overeating leads to extra weight on the joints; isolating and staying in bed can lead to depression and muscle atrophy; certain foods could lead to horrible intestinal reactions; pushing yourself too hard at the gym or PT can lead to injury and embarrassing ER visits. There are consequences for being out of balance. And for EDS, maintaining balance is always a goal.

DO: Practice mindfulness to be aware of what you are doing and not doing.

Again, if you are not aware, then you cannot make the best decisions for your body. Start with becoming aware by stopping and taking three deep breaths. Then say several times a day, "I am aware," and bring your awareness to what you are doing. How are you sitting, standing? What are you eating? How is your day structured? Is your day, life, and home helpful for your condition? Have you reached out for support for any overwhelming feelings you are having? Are you avoiding certain responsibilities to your health? Is there a slight pain somewhere in your body? I always listen to the smallest signals of pain, for that is where I have the greatest opportunity to change course and keep myself healthy and happy.

Recap:

Listen to your body. Embrace pain as a messenger. Become more aware. Practice mindfulness in everything you do. Ask your body questions. Listen. Then, honor yourself. Be connected to your body—which means stopping often, checking in, and sitting still. Eliminate distractions that distract you from yourself and keep things simple.

Suggested Affirmations:

Try saying these out loud:

> "I listen to my body."
> "I am listening."
> "I honor and listen to my body."
> "Thank you, pain, for telling me about that."
> "I am aware."

Suggested Prayer:

Use the Serenity Prayer as often as needed. While we may not be able to change our DNA or our condition, we can change our thoughts about it and our attitude. We may even find a few practical things we can change when we have some serenity.

> *"God, grant me the serenity to accept the things I*
> *cannot change,*
> *the courage to change the things I can,*
> *and wisdom to know the difference."*
> —The Serenity Prayer, author unknown

KEY #2

ADJUSTMENTS

"Aerodynamically the bumblebee shouldn't be able to fly, but the bumblebee doesn't know that so it goes on flying anyway."
—Mary Kay Ash

NEEDING SUPPORT
STEPPING INTO "THE SOLUTIONS" WITH THE RIGHT HELP

"Life is not about waiting for the storms to pass.
It's about learning how to dance in the rain."
—Vivian Greene

I couldn't do it alone. I had to put my pride aside and redefine what pride meant to me. I quickly learned that the only way to survive with EDS is with support. No matter how independent and self-sufficient I wanted to be, I now needed others. Then, I discovered the only way to thrive living with EDS is with good supports, a solid structure, and serious self-discipline. The longer that I lived with my condition, the more I ended up needing support with practically everything. This was a very humbling experience, and it became emotional for me. Every time I had to ask for help, I resisted it and ended up in some kind of sadness and tears. I missed out on being grateful for all the help because I always felt so much self-pity and defeat.

My list of supports that I needed to survive EDS and live a quality life became extensive. I needed supplement support with multi-vitamins and extra vitamin C. I needed support carrying things. I needed knee supports, neck supports, back supports, etc. I needed surgical supports. I also needed emotional support. I needed support in creating a strategy for survival. On some of my bad days, I needed support with keeping a positive attitude. I needed therapy support to face my diagnosis and prognosis. I needed support, even to go get support! The mixture of stubbornness, self-pity, and defeatism was not helpful but instead very harmful.

Pro Tip: Get help getting help (if you are stubborn or stuck).

Not having support meant increased anxiety for me. I noticed that the level of anxiety I was having always correlated with how much support I had for whatever health challenge was happening at the time. I learned that to curb my anxiety, I needed to ask for help: sometimes, a lot of help. Having people who knew about my condition and were reliable helpers for rides and listening mattered a great deal to me and reduced my stress. I worried less when I knew that someone "had my back." My problems arose when I tried to manage my condition without support. For a short time, I rebelliously practiced denial and attempted to forget that I had EDS and live like everyone else. . . only to hurt myself trying. Don't do this! Trying to do it alone led to injury and illness. My pride was often hurt when I hit a wall and found my limitations very, well, I guess I am saying... limiting.

I had another obstacle to getting support. It was the shame I carried deep inside about my condition. I was ashamed to be young and needing so much help. Daily, I had to release shame and offer myself forgiveness for feeling bad about myself. Truthfully, I was embarrassed to be me— because it meant I was fragile, compromised, delicate, and vulnerable. However, with the help of supportive people, I learned that fragility was a judgment I was placing on myself. And this type of self-judgment was harmful. See how important getting support is!?

I was learning who I was and getting answers year after year surviving with EDS. But I wasn't what the world of overachievers idolized. I wasn't what success was supposed to look like at my age. I wasn't a tough millennial warrior who fought, pushed through, and tackled life with fierceness, fire, and force. I was the opposite. Cautious, concerned, worried, fearful, and living life "low key" to avoid the spotlight and to avoid embarrassment, I didn't want to expose myself as a disabled person, and I wanted so badly to keep up with everyone else.

My other problem was that I was originally surrounded by unsupportive people who seemed to target a weak, kind, and caring person like myself. The problem with those people was that they weren't reliable and often criticized me for not being able to do whatever it was they wanted. As much as I loved a party, I couldn't party like them. These were the kind of people who used subtle forms of peer pressure to push their agenda on me. And I had a habit of caving under any pressure.

Sometimes, I tried to force myself to tag along to events they wanted, only to find myself exhausted and overextended from trying to keep up. If I had given myself permission and known my limits, I could have searched for people more my speed and pace, which would have supported me. However, I wasn't aware that I was being targeted for the simple fact that I so badly wanted to be like them. My jealousy of how normal people lived the fast life made me vulnerable. I was susceptible to toxic, pressuring-type people because I wanted a life that didn't belong to me. I wanted to be normal. I wanted to live a normal life. I wanted to do what normal teens and twenty- and thirty-year-olds did. I wanted to be like them. I just couldn't. I physically couldn't. I didn't know that I had EDS, and I certainly didn't know who I was back then. But I do remember not being able to keep up and feeling different.

When I finally reached the age of forty, I let a lot go and started designing a different life and vision for myself. A vision that revolved around who I am. I created a lifestyle that was supportive for me. This was when I stepped into "The Solutions" for myself and out of all my problems of trying to be like others. I started supporting myself. I started asking for support. I stopped shaming myself. I stopped hurting myself with "shoulds." I sought better surroundings. I supported myself with common sense, ergonomics, and logic. I supported myself with self-compassion, self-forgiveness, and self-understanding. I stopped blaming myself for the genes I was born with. I supported myself with self-love. And that made all the difference.

When professionals, doctors, and geneticists couldn't offer me a sustainable treatment or cure for my condition, I turned back to yoga for help with my health. This was a way that I could support myself safely when others didn't understand. Although yoga was classified as contraindicated, I believe that they had their advice incorrect. Stretching is not advisable for joints that are already too lax. Still, the other elements of yoga— the strengthening, breathing, being in the body, meditation and relaxation— were what my body desperately needed. To be as healthy as I could be, I learned to listen to the experts on some things and listen to myself for other things. I still maintained the recommended EDS Physical Therapy Routine and took long walks, but I listened to myself and stayed away from chiropractors and gravitated toward learning all I could about gentle yoga and vitamin supplementation.

Pro Tip: Don't seek out quick fixes (as they may be dangerous).
*Unless you are in an emergency situation and a medical doctor is trying to save your life.

I will recognize the inherent danger in trying to get support: while it may help, it can also harm. My trip to the chiropractor for pain relief showed me that. The neck tendon tear has followed me and haunted my craniocervical instability ever since. So, I had to be careful and cautious about what type of support I sought out. Even supplementation was harmful. Many times I was sick from vitamins and supplements meant to help. Through trial and error, I found some safe things that supported me. Sometimes getting support to deal with the fact that there are no solutions *is* the solution.

Self-Coaching Questions:

(Journal your answers for yourself.)

1. Where do you currently need support?
2. What supports have you tried that were harmful?
3. What supports have been recommended that you haven't tried?

ADJUSTING TO A NEW REALITY
AGING WITH EDS

"I can't change the direction of the wind,
but I can adjust my sails to always reach my
*   destination."*
-Jimmy Dean

Before my EDS diagnosis, before turning thirty-five, I felt somewhat normal, although deep down I knew I had always been different. I enjoyed the things most everyone else enjoyed at my age. I did many activities that everyone else did, although I instinctively veered away from sports. Thank God for instincts! I only felt a little sorry for myself back then. So what if I couldn't run a race? Who wanted to sweat that much anyways? But then, something changed as I aged. Was it the pregnancy hormones or just turning thirty? It may have been a combination of both. One thing I understood was that things got different as I aged.

Limitations, Restrictions, and More

I had a hard time adjusting to the new limitations and restrictions that I had to place on myself to avoid injury and illness. I had to make accommodations for my body that annoyed and aggravated me (and others who were trying to spend time with me). I had to let so many things go that I loved, including (and especially) going to the chiropractor for a quick fix. As much as I loved horseback riding, it was backbreaking, and I couldn't take the pressure on my spine or the impact. I would be painfully sore for a week after riding, reminding me of my limits. I had to stop going to the gym because I kept hurting myself using weight machines, and I would end up in the ER getting x-rays that showed nothing. My life had to change because life in the hospital wasn't appealing.

When I couldn't deny my invisible condition any longer, I began to grieve. Sadly, I allowed my grieving to turn into giving up. Sometimes I gave up. Since the hard workouts at physical therapy weren't solving my post-pregnancy issues after two full years of every lunge move/exercise imaginable, I decided it wasn't worth the embarrassment of being there at such a young age, walking around the elderly and frail. It felt like everyone was wondering why I was there. I certainly was! With a defeated attitude, I gave up on myself a time or two. When I received the diagnosis, I mistakenly quit because there was no cure for EDS, so why bother?

All the Wrong Reasons

Quitting out of anger, self-pity, and resentment felt good for a while; that is, until my body started to deteriorate further due to my lack of physical exercise. As a direct result, I then had new injuries to contend with—injuries from doing nothing. Weakness set in during my quitting phase, and that spelled disaster for my joints. Faced with new problems, I had to reconsider my position and attitude of "why bother?"

The Adjustment Process / Making Lists

If I wanted to be able to live independently, I had to adjust myself to my circumstances, my diagnosis, and the facts of aging with a connective tissue disorder. My older age had to mean new activities for me. To keep perspective, I began to list all the things that I instinctively knew that I couldn't do as a kid and began adding things that I now knew I couldn't do, like chiropractic adjustments and advanced yoga poses. I also knew I couldn't fall into despair and quit everything all together. To encourage myself, I had to begin to list the things that I could do and add new activities to that list. This new list included writing blogs and books, reading, taking a short drive, walking, coffee shop mediations, and volunteering to help little kids. Both lists had to grow. I had to adjust.

I noticed that when I adjusted, things became easier emotionally. I had more optimism when I looked at the list of things I could do. The "Can Do" list included things that I loved. My "Can't Do Anymore" list included things that I used to love. I learned to love the memory of those activities and let those chapters close as any wise and aging person would do. I had to be sure to balance the memories of things past with the anticipation of things to enjoy. I still thought of them fondly but no longer focused on that list. I stopped entertaining self-pity this way. Thus, I opened up new chapters just waiting to be written.

Suggested Self-Coaching / Journaling Assignment:

1. Make a list of things you "Can't Do Any Longer" (and cherish those beautiful memories)
2. Make a list of things you "Can Do and Enjoy" (try to do one a day)
3. Note: Focus on the "Can Do" list. Think of the "Can't Do" list as an exercise in self-discipline, self-control, and self-compassion for any grieving that needs to take place.

KEY #3

ACKNOWLEDGEMENT

"Not everything that is faced can be changed, but nothing can be changed until it is faced."
—James Baldwin

ACKNOWLEDGEMENT

"Knowledge is in the end based on acknowledgement."
—Ludwig Wittgenstein

I had to acknowledge myself. I had to accept and admit the existence of this truth. I have EDS.

This was another emotional step for me. Even though I didn't want it to be so, it was. While seemingly simple, this wasn't always easy. Nor was it clear that I had slipped back into denial or ignorance again. Regressing to pre-diagnosis thoughts and ways of living were part of my steps forward. Usually, an injury or profound illness would help me acknowledge EDS again—if I had temporarily forgotten. To survive, I had to recognize that I was different and oftentimes at a disadvantage, healthwise and physically, from my peers. This was always emotional for me.

I also had to acknowledge the existence of research and findings on EDS's many types and aspects. Spending time reviewing the already-published information and storing it in my mind (as helpful data) allowed me to directly acknowledge that science was on the frontier of making this DNA discovery and learning how to help. Doctors were having new insights into the matter. They were taking a new interest in the rare. New comorbidities were being linked, and new medicines were available. Even a few moms were publishing their own EDS protocol to keep their kids healthy and get them up out of wheelchairs. Everyone on the front line of this disorder was offering insight.

The Limits and Limitations

It was difficult to acknowledge that the global medical community and researchers had limitations on what they knew about this rare syndrome and how to treat it. I expected more from doctors than they had to give. I expected us to be further along with scientific discoveries than we were. I expected answers when I reached certain specialties like orthopedics, only to find that they were clueless. I expected a protocol to avoid surgery when I reached the neurosurgeon who saw more desperate, critical EDS patients than anyone else. I expected solid answers to tests and results. These expectations led me to so much disappointment and years of search-and-fail missions. We didn't know what we didn't know.

Besides acknowledging my past medical history, I had to acknowledge where I was at and what condition I was living with. I had to acknowledge my limits daily, weekly, monthly, yearly. On the flip side, to get my mind off a negative track, I had to acknowledge my blessings. For all the unlucky DNA strands I inherited, I also was lucky to have lived to forty. I was blessed to have a child and create a manageable life for myself and my condition. As one of my life-saving surgeons said, "You have more in common with the average person than differences." I always hung onto that statement. It felt like I had to rely on normal things about me to see me through healing and recovery. And life, for that matter!

> *"Real life isn't always going to be perfect or go our way, but the recurring acknowledgement of what is working in our lives can help us not only to survive but surmount our difficulties."*
> —Sarah Ban Breathnach

Prior to the second neck injury, which exacerbated my CCI, I had insisted on living a normal life. I wanted to push through my limitations and keep up with the rat race of society. I had a strong will, determination, and passion for living. My forceful insistence led me to early burnout and lots of injuries and ended in broken self-esteem. It took years of prying apart my life and my decisions to see that I had inadvertently tied my self-worth and self-esteem to what I could do and accomplish in this world. I craved worldly success and centered my existence around it. It took many health crises to rearrange my priorities and give myself a sweet and simple life. Success had to be redefined for me to stop making myself feel bad about life.

The Paradox of Life

I had to acknowledge all the paradoxes that I was living with. Everything was both. I had to do, but not do too much. I had to rest, and yet I had to work to keep up my strength. I had to work, but not at something that was too stressful, too hard, or that put me at risk. I had to get medical help but not rely on it 100% to live. I had to go all-natural, and then sometimes not. I had to be in the hospital, and be out of the hospital. I had to take medicines, but not all the time and not too much. I used wisdom and acknowledged that some doctors were right and some were very, very wrong. I had to listen and obey, and sometimes I had to defy and get multiple second opinions. I had to go for testing and opt-out of other types of testing. I had to sort through all the helpful and non-helpful things (medication, advice, supplements, natural therapies) in relation to EDS. I had to discover the healthy choices for my condition. I sometimes was able to enjoy normal activities, and other times I had to make a ton of alterations. I had to push myself, but not. I had to make adjustments to my daily tasks, as well as my thinking.

> *"What seems to us as bitter trials are often*
> *blessings in disguise."*
> —Oscar Wilde

EDS WAS A CURSE AND A BLESSING. I had to live it both ways. The reality was both. To live a balanced life, to be balanced in my mind... I had to acknowledge both or be tipped into the darkness of depression or the bliss of ignorance. I didn't want to keep blaming everything on bad luck like my younger brother did. It only led to more bad luck. I once told him that we create our own good luck, but he could not receive that message the loving way it was intended. I hoped to give him the gift of knowing that he had the power of choice when he felt so powerless. Undiagnosed EDS ruined his life and left him crippled for most of it. It wasn't just his back that was completely broken; it was his self-esteem. Self-pity broke him too. Being at a disadvantage, with disadvantages to begin with, was so sad to witness. I loved him so much but was unable to fix his life for him.

To pull out of any depressions or self-pity, I had to acknowledge the gifts of EDS. It physically gave me abilities that others did not have. I had to hear my truth rise up, allow it to become really strong, and get really good at listening. With lots of alone time, I discovered that I often had the answers for myself. I feel like I became the most compassionate, sympathetic, and empathetic person I knew. There surely was a gift in that. The pain, the suffering, the agony, the constant medical uncertainty helped me meet those dying with cancer and other ailments with so much more care, concern, and understanding. It made me a great person to share a burden with. Even more so, I became very experienced/ knowledgeable about everything health and medical—more so than the average person. I could always provide insight into courses of treatment and next steps to those around me because I had already gone the route myself. Perhaps others benefited from my suffering and hard-earned-through-sickness knowledge. I hope so.

Without true, living acknowledgement that I had this rare syndrome, I was living a lie. I was lying to myself when I wouldn't accept it. To hide it, I was falsely trying to be like the majority of typical people. While blending in can be helpful and allow me to fit into most circumstances, it also caused me to blend in too well. Some disabilities aren't visible at all. I had to acknowledge that. And people who lack empathy or understanding simply couldn't acknowledge it. So it was really important that I did this step for myself. I never got caught in the trap of hoping my family would acknowledge it. I never waited for their acknowledgement of my condition. I watched how year after year, they stumbled through life with health challenges, unwilling to acknowledge that they too had this condition. I felt sorry for them and lucky that I was able to acknowledge myself. This step helped me make so many better decisions—ones that were life-saving and life-serving.

> *"In the depth of winter, I finally learned that*
> *within me there lay an invincible summer."*
> —Albert Camus

Self-Reflection Questions:

1. Where do you do too much?
2. Where do you not do enough?
3. What do you need to acknowledge about your EDS?
4. What do you need to acknowledge about yourself?
5. What are you afraid to acknowledge?
6. What goodness about your life can you acknowledge?

(Journal your thoughts and feelings.)

KEY #4

ACTION*

*"If we wait until we're ready,
we'll be waiting for the rest of our lives."*
—Lemony Snicket

*Wise counsel was given to me that Acceptance needs to come before Action. Please keep this in mind as you continue reading. My reasoning for this particular order is that it took me a long time to accept my EDS diagnosis, which held me back from taking care of myself. I needed to still be practicing good self-care while my emotions caught up with the reality of my genetic condition.

ACTION
RAISING AWARENESS AND ADVOCACY

*"To trust in your own aliveness, in your own
    ability to sustain and be sustained - there are
    times when there is no greater act of
    defiance."*
—Jessica Fechtor

Sometimes it is incumbent upon us to take necessary action. It might be to undergo surgery, partake in a physical therapy program designed for EDS, or something else. The action we take can vary from writing blogs or letters to hospitals, creating communities, and being part of the voice of a group, to practicing self-compassion and taking a walk. Whatever we do, it has to be mindful, and we have to do it consciously. Conscious choices lead to better outcomes.

The Importance of Goals

To stay motivated to act and follow-through, I had to create goals. I made several small goals that were attainable and larger goals to work towards. I would set a goal of walking the track three times a day and then push it to six. I would make a goal of seven minutes of strengthening yoga on the mat, and push it to ten minutes to improve gradually. I also set goals to get more sleep and go to bed earlier. I had health goals of eating salmon three times a week for breakfast. All these goals had me taking action in the right direction. These small steps added up. I was contributing to a health bank account. It was important for me to design my own goals because I had to be ready, willing, and able to make them and meet them. This helped boost my self-esteem. Each effort toward a goal was an esteemable act. Even cleaning goals became uplifters while I was stuck home with MCAS flares or the multitude of EDS restrictions. Organizing my closets, paperwork and apartment gave me such a boost, just like exercise boosts endorphins. I needed as many natural remedies for my malady as I could get.

> *"If disabled people were truly heard, an explosion*
> *of knowledge of the human body and psyche*
> *would take place."*
> —Susan Wendell

The Importance of Groups

When COVID-19 hit the U.S., all of my group exercise classes, self-help study gatherings, and spiritual meetings came to an abrupt halt. The absence of these groups (and subsequent understandable mini-depression) demonstrated how important the group atmosphere and sharing were to my life. Going to those meetings was the best action that I took. Safe healing groups boost good hormones in the body and I dearly missed them. I found ways to join online groups and forums to stay connected. I also found phone meetings and other meetings to attend. Attending meetings and groups helped pull me out of isolation. It connected me to others on levels that I could reach. I may not be able to run a marathon with them, but I could sit for an hour and explore topics like grief and healing. Finding new groups and ones that fit me was one of the pillars of my life and still is. Speaking up (and speaking out) helped me and other members.

DO: Create your own list of "solutions" and follow through with your goals.

See the back of the book for a list of My Solutions for helpful suggestions.

The Act of Self-Compassion

With EDS, I needed heaps of self-compassion to get me through life. Others, who didn't suffer as often nor as much, simply couldn't provide me with the type of empathy I needed to survive emotionally. I needed compassion for all the tremendous amounts of pain and suffering I had endured from not only my condition, but from the unsympathetic medical doctors I met along the way. I had to give myself approval on a daily basis. These self-approval statements meant the world to my self-esteem. "I love and approve of myself." "I accept myself the way I am." "I still give myself love when others can't."

The Gift of Movement

I took actions to move my body and push myself to at least walk daily, which spared me some issues. I often had to challenge myself to include hills and different things that could strengthen my core muscles. I had to move my body to maintain my muscle mass in the face of EDS. The few times that I had to be on bed rest showed me how serious the implications for not moving could be. A few times of binge-watching Netflix showed me how sitting for extended periods of time can really weaken my neck and back. I had to take action daily. I had to move my body uphill, up stairs, up to the rubber track. These actions benefited me tremendously when PT was canceled due to COVID-19.

> *It's so important to keep moving and don't buy*
> *into the myth. I say do anything you feel like*
> *as long as you don't hurt yourself or hurt*
> *anyone else. And things don't stop working*
> *in your body or your mind.*
> —Florence Henderson

The Gift of Stillness

Not teaching yoga classes for a year really showed in my body. I was weaker, prone to more flares, and overall not as able and stable and healthy as when teaching was part of my regular week. Each class that I taught, even gentle yoga, was an investment in my health. The lack of all these regular, routine things really makes my EDS worse. It was up to me to find a way to supplement. I became what I call the "Two-walks-a-day woman." While some of my walks were power-packed to discharge energy and anxiety, most were strolls in nature to clear or prep my mind. The mind-body connection was so powerful that my meditations were most effective after a long walk, or midway. I found a favorite meditation bench or two that I stopped at mid-walk to quiet my thoughts and just be. The act of having a regular meditation practice has been advised by gurus and therapists as well as modern-day sciences. Sleep and meditation were two types of stillness that benefited my EDS. All other "slacking" was harmful.

When it felt like there was nothing I could do about my current situation, I often realized the best I could do was offer the next generation a solid foundation to stand on. Those who were raising awareness, creating groups, and participating in or starting research gave me causes that I could get behind and contribute to. Giving a vial of blood to be part of a study felt like the right course of action. I wanted to be part of the solution as much as I was dealing with all the problems.

I also had to advocate for myself and others. Sometimes offering my name and contact information to a younger person struggling with EDS was the best I could do. Providing a listening ear was an act of mercy for the souls of EDS sufferers. I made it a daily mission to reach out and provide comfort, concern, and care. This meant the world to those with EDS who had no one local to connect with.

> *"There is no magic cure, no making it all go away forever. There are only small steps upward; an easier day, an unexpected laugh, a mirror that doesn't matter anymore."*
> —Laurie Halse Anderson

I also had to speak up to doctors and give them educational resources. I had to be prepared for every appointment to hand them valuable information linking two rare syndromes via medical journals or print-outs explaining complications. I went in with a file instead of relying on them to know.

Follow Up and Seek The Experts

It was important for me to follow up and keep my appointments with doctors. Oftentimes I was so fatigued and disillusioned that I saw no point in going to these follow-up appointments. Meeting local doctors with no experience with EDS often led me to despair and made me resist going to more doctors in the same field. However, when I would find that one helpful physician who had experience, it would boost my belief in modern medicine. When I began following up with specialists in all departments, I gained knowledge and specifics along the way that helped me pick which medicines might work. All the follow-up appointments helped me pinpoint my problems, mostly by ruling out other diseases. I cannot stress the importance of following up with doctors and getting a good understanding of your condition or conditions. Some doctors that I thought would be a waste of time were later life-saving. Some tests that I thought would reveal nothing revealed something major. I found answers in the strangest of medical appointments. I learned to just keep my principle in place of following up, no matter how discouraged I felt.

> *"If you desire to make a difference in the world,*
> *you must be different from the world."*
> —Elaine Dalton

Self-Reflection Questions:

1. What action do you need to take for yourself?
2. What actions can you take for others with EDS?
3. How can you create a safe exercise plan?
4. How can you create healthy habits?
5. How can you incorporate meditation into your life?

6. What goal can you set for yourself?
7. What group can you join?

KEY #5

ACCEPTANCE*

"Why fit in when you were born to stand out?"
—Dr Seuss

*Needed for inner peace

ACCEPTANCE

"You remain what you are."
—Flannery O'Connor,
Everything That Rises Must Converge

I had survived many near-death experiences—three of which pushed me to write this book. I had survived infections and the torture of year's worth of medical PTSD. I had finally recognized that my EDS/MCAS combo was certainly the underlying cause for all the episodes I faced. I had finally altered my life and reformed my thinking on how to go about living with EDS. It took years to reach a level of acceptance that allowed me to live in peace. There were often levels of acceptance that I hadn't reached but still strived for. For example, how could scientists and geneticists not find the hEDS or MCAS gene yet? I had to learn to live "in the mystery" which became the art of acceptance. I would not only always live with uncertainty but also without so many much-needed answers.

Do: Learn to live in the mystery.

The Anger That Came

Somehow, having EDS felt completely unfair to me. During those self-pity parties, I was taking my condition personally. This was really an impersonal issue. It wasn't done to me on purpose. Neither my mother nor father had any clue. Perhaps if others in my family had gotten diagnosed and were open about this, I would have more easily accepted my unfortunate circumstances. But I felt like the only one suffering and willing to investigate for an underlying cause. I had no paved road to follow, only the task of trying to pave some of this rough/bumpy-as-all-heck road for my child. I had to allow room for my anger but not let it consume me. I accepted that anger was a normal human emotion. What I could do was let it fuel me into doing something constructive instead of hating EDS and hating myself.

The Other Emotions

I had to process all the anger, grief, and sadness over my situation to reach acceptance. I acknowledged my own limited human existence. It reminded me of my cigarette-smoking devout Catholic grandmother (a lung cancer patient) always defending herself by saying: "We are all going to die of something!" She was right of course. However, I didn't want to contribute to my own death. I wanted to contribute to a healthy life full of adventures, fun, joy, and experiences. Mostly, I wanted to usher my daughter through childhood and see her reach adulthood safe and sound. I didn't want to leave her behind motherless. Nor did I want to leave her with this condition and no guidance or emotional support. I had to accept that I would die, but how or when—I felt sometimes like I might have a small or large say. Other times, when things were medically beyond my control, I found peace in accepting that I may die "young." I learned to tell myself that I would just be in heaven at a younger age. Somehow, that rephrasing helped me immensely to accept the inevitable. The less I struggled with reality and truth, the more at ease I was with EDS.

Being My Own Primary Care Doctor

I knew that I needed my body to stay in one piece. I couldn't fracture myself anymore with modern medical remedies. I needed to respect the philosophy of "wholism." I was a functioning organism struggling with mostly all my parts. It was vital for me to accept that I couldn't kill my liver to save my heart, and I couldn't take pain meds to stop the important messages from getting through. I had to accept that this (pain and problems) was my plight. I was and would be always dealing with medical stuff. Always dealing with pain. Always dealing with EDS. Always navigating the commodities. Always a slave to my MCAS.

I had to accept that I would never find the perfect doctor to take on me as a whole person with all my issues. I wanted a parent figure to watch over me and tell me what to do. I had to accept that this wasn't available. Maybe someday there would be connective tissue disorder clinics in each city. Maybe someday doctors would call their patients back and check on them. But it wasn't happening now. I had to accept this responsibility for myself even though I wasn't a doctor and was new to all of this physiology and genetics stuff. I accepted the position because no one else would. No one was even qualified. Not even me.

I accepted that I had to stop trying to make this permanent condition go away or find a cure. I had to accept that this would just be case management and sometimes comfort measures. I once had a flare of MCAS so bad that I called my doctor and asked for "end of life care." Being stuck in a hospital bed with my joints all falling out of place, in level 9 (out of 10) pain day and night, was not something I could live with. I wanted a dignified and pain-free escape from life and suffering. That's about the time doctors would take out the big guns for me, like prednisone, and coax me back to life.

I had to accept the emotional rollercoaster—the ups and downs, the victories and defeats. My time had to be spent on designing a life that would be sustainable for me and allow me the most freedom. I had to accept that my previous freedoms were revoked with injuries. That pushed me to find and create new ways to flourish. Oftentimes, I felt like the only ones who could understand this struggle to survive were other severe EDSers, MCASers, or terminal cancer patients. Keeping a healthy perspective, I could identify with others but not compare.

> *"Don't compare yourself with anyone in this world. If you do so you are insulting yourself."*
> —Bill Gates

We Are Not the ONLY Ones

Out of curiosity about genetics, I began learning about other rare genetic disorders, and noted how one single "oops" gene could set people up for so many problems. As full-functioning humans we need thousands of working parts to work in order to live a healthy, happy life. When I saw other rare syndromes in my research, it helped me gain perspective on my own and often catapulted me into gratitude for what I felt cursed with. My curse would be considered a blessing compared to some of these other genetic situations. I saw many gene-sufferers being born without arms or legs! That helped me see that even though my limbs struggled and were painful—at least I had them! A wider view of genetic issues helped me to accept my own with grace and gratitude.

DO: Get a bigger view of genetics to find your gratitude.

Failing on the Way to Success

I had to accept the failures with my success. Acceptance was the only way of having peace with my condition. Fighting it, arguing against it, ignoring it, dodging it, denying it—all were sure ways to lose my precious energy and just drove me around in a great big circle back to myself. Those were trips to nowhere. I found a hundred ways not to think about EDS for the sake of my mental health.

Acceptance also opened me up to possibilities. "I have EDS... now what?" became the best question for me to ask when facing my day and creating goals for my life. I embraced my diagnoses and had to live accordingly. I no longer could live while working against myself in order to achieve success. I had to take this step of acceptance whole-heartedly.

> *"We should celebrate diversity–the world*
> *would be*
> *poorer and life duller if we were all the same."*
> —Neil Milliken

Nature's Design?

Often, I marveled at nature's genius. There were so many plants and animals designed so uniquely for various reasons. I often thought of myself like the bendy willow tree in the midst of mighty strong oaks. I, like the willow tree, needed more water than most and learned to bend in the wind and not break. Whereas the oak tree can grow strong and hold steady during a storm, my DNA had adapted someone to flow and not fight. I didn't have much push-back to give from my flexible body, so I was forced to learn how to flow with the blows. I made a decision one day to not fight my diagnosis of EDS, and that made all the difference.

Most of all, acceptance allowed me to love myself and my design. I stopped looking at myself as a broken person or a mistake. I had to look back on my forty years and see my contributions to society, women, and the world. I had to push past perfectionism and a perfectionist culture to be able to do this. Perfectionism held no room for me. Acceptance did.

> *"It's not our disabilities, it's our abilities that*
> *count."*
> —Chris Burke

What I Didn't Know = the Many Contraindications

To my error, I made the mistake of trying horseback riding lessons when I turned eighteen. I dearly loved horses and always dreamed of riding, but couldn't afford it while growing up. I started, only to learn that the impact of a horse walking, trotting or galloping was crushing and damaging to my spine. After all those sore experiences and attempts, I had to give up. But I never gave up loving horses. The brutal dry hard land made it clear to me that I belonged in the water. I had to let that dream die and accept that this form of exercise was not a right fit. The bruises on my calves reminded me week after week of the problem with impact and strain on my body. During one group lesson, we were asked to turn around in the saddle to improve our confidence and balance. Because I was a late starter, I was with much younger kids learning to ride. A rebellious boy decided to play and remain backwards, to the annoyance of the instructor. I shouted something like, "Hey, kid, you don't want to end up like Superman," referring to the horse injury sustained by the famous actor that played him. I was hoping that he would realize that he was not invincible or beyond getting hurt on a horse. The instructor solemnly, sadly remarked that the actor often rode at these stables and my comment hurt. I was shocked and embarrassed. I had never met a movie star before and classified them as immortal people somewhere in Hollywood. I apologized, of course, out of sincere respect for the actor. What I really needed to say was that I was not Superwoman. That I could not do it all and was subject to getting hurt. Little did I know that 20 years later, I would be needing a wheelchair too.

Some Laughter Led to Some Acceptance

Over the years, I learned that even movie stars and famous people have/face incredible health challenges. Lucky for us more of them are being open about their struggles and not just putting on a perfect smile for the cameras. I accepted that I just had to love horses from a distance and take up swimming. That's not to say that I didn't attempt surfing in California, only to learn that drowning was also not a fun form of exercise! I learned that when I could laugh at myself and the issues that plagued me from EDS and MCAS, I had reached a higher level of acceptance. Light-hearted laughter (not sarcasm, nor jokes at my expense) was really what showed me my progress with acceptance. I learned that I was powerless over so many things. I admitted that. I also learned that I could influence others and had the power to make choices large and small. However, the powerlessness over reality led to more acceptance for me.

> *"A sense of humor is a major defense against*
> *minor troubles."*
> — Mignon McLaughlin

I often felt like a tired hero on a hero's journey while facing EDS and MCAS. I had to rescue myself from bad medical experiences, doctors who didn't know, and the world that couldn't visibly or easily see my struggle. I learned to save myself from self-pity as much as from doctor's mistakes and misdiagnoses. It sometimes took herculean efforts to overcome my fears of medicine, trying new things, or trusting doctors who turned out to be reliable. If we are all on a hero's journey, then we must save ourselves before we can save others. I accepted this mission and grew gradually into the strength of spirit that I needed to live and thrive with EDS.

> *"A hero is an ordinary individual who finds*
> *strength to preserve and endure in spite of*
> *overwhelming obstacles."*
> —Christopher Reeve (1952-2004)

Self-Reflection Questions:

1. What have you not accepted?
2. Where do you not have peace?
3. What does acceptance mean for you?
4. Write 10 things you are grateful for.

BONUS #6

ACCOMODATIONS

"A bend in the road is not the end of the road.
Unless you fail to make the turn."
—Helen Keller

ACCOMMODATIONS
BEING HIGH MAINTENANCE

*"You may encounter many defeats, but you must
not be defeated. In fact, it may be necessary
to encounter the defeats, so you can know
who you are, what you can rise from, how
you can still come out of it."*
— Maya Angelou

If pregnancy and childbirth didn't kill me, if a neck adjustment at the chiropractor didn't kill me, if craniocervical instability, and Mast Cell Activation Disorder flare-ups didn't kill me, then I was encountering many defeats, yet not being defeated.

I realized very early that my body was like a high-maintenance car. It needed a lot of oil and downtime ("garage time"). It took years to learn how to drive my body and how to steer clear of pain and problems. Sometimes it felt like walking a tightrope or driving on a narrow one-lane road around mountains abutted against steep cliffs. It was like, one wrong move could create a crash or mean the end. It was incredibly frustrating to always have to be "watching out" for things.

Self-Preservation / Self-Protection / Self-Care

I had to watch the food I ate to ensure I didn't overload my body with sugar or histamine. I had to watch how much weight I put on each joint so that I didn't tear a ligament or rupture a tendon. I had to watch out for when I got extremely fatigued and needed to rest, or else risk collapse and loss of consciousness. I had to watch out for doctors that treated this zebra like a regular horse and dismissed my claims that I am different. I had to watch out and watch my back.

DO: Stay True to Your DNA

This led me to make many permanent, new lifestyle changes. I had to accommodate all my needs for movement, rest, food sensitivities, medicine issues, etc. When sleeping in a bed is so painful and such a nightly problem, you know that you will have to make daytime accommodations too. I often had to buy different types of chairs and rotate them just to type and spend time at the computer. Getting comfortable took hours and was exhausting. It was no wonder why I fidgeted so much as a child. I simply could not sit still, or I had joint pain. This is why muscle fatigue became a real thing.

To thrive, I had to always accommodate my EDS. This meant that I was aware, and that I acknowledged and accepted my disorder and prognosis. I often felt frustrated with how scaled back my life became. How I had to let go of certain things I enjoyed with every new issue or injury. I had to accommodate myself as a disabled person when most people and places couldn't or wouldn't. This became a full-time job for me. I had to design my life to fit my EDS instead of waiting for someone to accommodate my disability.

It took so much therapy and many self-worth exercises for me to admit to being disabled. If it weren't for CCI, I probably would have kept pushing and punishing my body to live an average high-paced modern lifestyle. It felt more like admitting defeat than accepting my condition. I cried and often doubted my disability, only to have a day or month spent in a hospital bed or wheelchair to wake me out of my denial again. I knew that no employer could grant this many sick days and this much time off. Plus, my "health stuff" took priority over an employer, so pretending that I could keep working full-time wasn't feasible.

With the COVID-19 pandemic at my heels, I had to take precautions around others since they refused to do so. To me, the pandemic really separated those who care about others from those who don't. This meant I had to isolate myself to the max. It was tough because I had already given up most of my original dreams and life to the last round of injuries, only to tighten and further restrict my life.

However, I had to do what was necessary for me to survive. My safety came first over the non-maskers' and anti-vaxxers' loud, obnoxious, and misled voices. I knew that I had too much trouble with common colds and regular infections to deal with being exposed to a virus that can drop healthy grown men. I had to play it smart and play it safe. I sequestered and accommodated myself.

I embraced technology and what it could give me for entertainment, distraction, and education. I found creative solutions to my need to get away and bought a new camper/trailer. I had to find ways around mold exposure and COVID-19 exposure that could give me a rich, fun, interesting and exciting life—around the parameters of my EDS/MCAS combo.

I remember the day that I bought my first power-lift recliner at age thirty-nine (not something I thought I would need until I was elderly). It gave me the freedom to sit for hours and be upright. I faced it toward my window that overlooked downtown. It helped me feel part of my community even though I had to maintain being very separate.

I found outdoor activities for my child so that we could both enjoy her childhood. I found new rubber walking tracks to walk that were easier on my knees and joints and not too far away from the EMTs if I needed help. We found clean heated pools to enjoy and local things to explore because I couldn't drive too far in a hard neck brace. I packed a purse that might as well have been a suitcase of items and medicines to survive my conditions (and to be prepared if I somehow ended up in the hospital).

I learned to make appointments in the morning, or request phone or video appointments. I learned to adjust and make these accommodations for myself. The few people who understood my disorder were kind and understanding when I asked for help. The rest of the world didn't understand. I often had to accommodate for that.

Learning to prioritize myself and my safety helped me enjoy life and keep on living with EDS. Trying to force myself to be like everyone else led to failure, injury, and disappointment. Accommodating myself is how I truly lived successfully with EDS. Knowing myself, building on experiences, learning the lessons of others with EDS, all gave me the strength to advocate and ask when I needed to. I learned there was no shame with EDS.

Keeping my disorder hidden and not being honest about what I needed often led to failure. By making accommodations, I met new levels of success. Whereas some days, I would be pushing a wheelchair three times around the track due to a flare-up, others I would run half a lap and go around six times wheelchair free. What mattered was that I accommodated what my body needed. Some days were spent resting, others were spent moving. My goal was to have a balance of both on each day. But I never put myself down for what I could and couldn't do. I often struggled to write chapters, remember where I left off, or get jobs completed. But I remembered that I had to accommodate my EDS along the way. I was facing much harder things than the average person to get my story out there.

Self-Reflection Questions:

1. What shame can you release?
2. What accommodations do you need to make for yourself?

MY SOLUTIONS LIST

Self-acceptance
Self-preservation
Safe-guarding
Self-approval
Self-discipline
Self-compassion

Kindness
Asking for help
Sharing my burden/pain
Talking to a caring friend
Attending a group meeting

Prayer
Meditation
Gentle yoga
Guided relaxation
Nature
Long walks
Short walks

Naps
Sleep (Night-time, nine hours)
Poetry
Inspirational talks
Uplifting books
Spiritual retreats
Fasting
Write/Blog
Distractions (Netflix, movies, games)
Education (learning and reading about EDS)
TED TALKS
Stand-up comedy

Self-love
Good friends
A Church community
Attending local events
Live music
Visits to lakes, waterfalls, oceans, mountains

Make your own list of self-care solutions:

_____
_____
_____
_____
_____
_____

7-DAY SELF-STARTER/SELF-LOVE CHECKLIST PLAN

"It's the repetition of affirmations that leads to belief. And once that belief becomes a deep conviction, things begin to happen."
—Muhammad Ali

Need to get out of a slump?
Feeling alone, tired, and just plain down from living with EDS?
Want to get moving and feel better?

This is a 7-DAY suggested self-help/self-love list that can be used as a guide for you to create a lifestyle and daily wellness plan for thriving with EDS. The habit/practice of making daily lists—to accomplish tasks, goals, and stay on track—is invaluable. Use this suggested list, check the box, or cross things off as you complete them. Feel free to add to these lists and subtract things that don't fit your day.

DO: Make daily lists.

Be bold and hold yourself accountable by tearing off or printing out these lists to keep them handy in your kitchen or nearby. Pick a color pen, marker, or crayon to mark each item completed. Feel free to modify or add to this list to suit your needs or accommodate your situation. Think of this as a daily challenge—and challenge yourself to come out better each day. You may find these lists easy or hard depending on where you are at and what you are struggling with, so I encourage you to get creative and swap things out. Sometimes we come up with our best solutions and self-loving acts for ourselves. Know that, completing each of these lists is an esteemable act. Plus, you made it one more day living with EDS.

Hopefully, at the end of 7 days, you will feel energized, inspired, changed, and with a better outlook on life. Having a plan and following through can help you feel accomplished and successful in something. (Even if you are successful in just starting.) This forward momentum can help us to get unstuck. Think of each day, each "Key", as a way to unlock yourself and open new doors in your thinking and your life. I invite you to document and share your progress with the private FB group to keep us connected as a way to emotionally support your efforts.

DO: Designate a daily journal to list your gratitudes and write your thoughts/feelings.

CHALLENGE ACCEPTED?

(Start with Day #1)
Good for you and good luck!

DAY #1
AWARENESS

Today we are starting by focusing on our basic self-care needs and looking for what direction we would like our energy to take.

> *"The difference between those who fail and those who succeed is largely perseverance. Never quit."*
> —Charles Schwab

- Make goals. Write them down. *Forward thinking can help with setting a positive focus. Start by journaling and setting some goals. You can set big or small goals. (I like to make yearly goals to see where I am headed. Make daily or monthly goals for more manageability.)*
- Take a 10-minute walk (or any available exercise). Time yourself.
- Do 5 minutes of seated meditation after the walk (set a phone timer). Just breathe and try to settle your mind, body and spirit. (You can use music if needed.)
- Journal (Answer this question: "What is it I need?") Sit with the question for however long it takes to get a few answers.

This is best done after walking, after meditating…. You can bring this along for your walk.)
- Follow up by making a needed doctor's appointment.
- Read 1 thing that's uplifting.
- Listen to soothing music.
- Write 3 things you are grateful for.
- Go outside for 30 minutes somewhere beautiful.
- Call 1 friend to say "Hi."

Write about Key #1 – Awareness:

What are you aware of?

_____

_____

_____

_____

_____

_____

_____

_____

Bonus Work: Post on the FB group that you finished Day #1 of the challenge. Write your insights.

⇒**Skim over Day #2 to see what you need to plan for.**

DAY #2

ADJUSTING

"Concentrate on things your disability doesn't prevent you doing well, and don't regret the things it interferes with. Don't be disabled in spirit as well as physically."
—Stephen Hawking

- Write 3 things you are grateful for.
- Take a 15-minute walk.
- Do 5 minutes of meditation.
- Listen to 1 favorite song.
- Post online a compassionate response to someone struggling or send a Get Well note to a friend.
- Go outside for 30–60 minutes and take 3 deep breaths (even if it's raining).
- Read 1 chapter of a book (it can be a novel).
- Search for support groups that you can attend, call into or Zoom.
- Clean out a desk, shelf or drawer.
- Call a friend to say "Hello." (Ask how they are.)

Write about Key #2 – Adjustments:

What adjustments do you need to make in your life?

_____

_____

_____

_____

_____

_____

_____

_____

Bonus Work: Post on the FB group that you finished Day #2 of the challenge: write your insights.

⇒**Skim over Day #3 to see what you need to plan for.**

DAY #3
ACKNOWLEDGEMENT

"Being challenged in life is inevitable, being defeated is optional."
—Roger Crawford

- Do a 5-minute seated meditation (find a comfortable spot).
- Write down 5 things you are grateful for.
- Take a 15–30 minute walk somewhere new.
- Listen to 2 songs from 2 different genres.
- Schedule a free consultation call with a life-coach, or therapist.
- Buy a new item of clothing.
- Call or text a friend to say hi and how much you appreciate them.
- Listen to an uplifting TED talk.
- Read 1 chapter of a book.
- Eat something healthy.

Write about Key #3 – Acknowledgement

What do you need to acknowledge?

_____
_____
_____
_____
_____
_____
_____
_____

Bonus Work: Post on the FB group that you finished Day #3 of the challenge: write your insights.

⇒**Skim over Day #4 to see what you need to plan for.**

DAY #4
ACTION

"Continuous effort—not strength or intelligence —is the key to unlocking your potential."
—Winston Churchil

- Walk 30 minutes.
- 7-minute meditation
- Meet with a therapist, support group, counselor, or friend.
- Read 1 chapter of a book.
- Sit outside for 30 minutes.
- Play a song and dance to it (seated, standing).
- Eat something healthy.
- Take your vitamins or prescriptions needed.
- Do water therapy (take a shower, or bath, or go for a swim).
- Watch an inspiring movie.

Write about Key #4 Action:

What actions do you need to take?

_____

_____

_____

_____

_____

_____

_____

_____

Bonus Work: Post on the FB group that you finished Day #4 of the Self-Love/ Self-Starter Challenge: write your insights.

⇒**Skim over Day #5 to see what you need to plan for.**

DAY #5
ACCEPTANCE

"Acceptance doesn't mean resignation. It means understanding that something is what it is and there's going to be a way through it."
—Michael J. Fox

- Make up a helpful mantra. ("I am getting better and better, every day in every way.")
- Write down 10 things you are grateful for.
- Take a 5-30 minute walk.
- Sit somewhere new outdoors.
- Visit a monument, statue or church.
- Meet with a friend, therapist, or counselor and talk about your struggles.
- Read 1 chapter of a book.
- Take your vitamins or prescriptions.
- Eat something healthy.
- Read a famous quote or poem.

Write about Key #5 – Acceptance:

What can you accept? Or learn to accept?

_____
_____
_____
_____
_____
_____
_____
_____

Bonus Work: Post on the FB group that you finished Day #5 of the Self-Love Starter Challenge: write your insights.

⇒**Skim over Day #6 to see what you need to plan for.**

DAY #6

ACCOMMODATIONS

*"These days the technology can solve our
problems and then some. Solutions may not
only erase physical or mental deficits but
leave patients better off than 'able-bodied'
folks. The person who has a disability today
may have a superability tomorrow."*
—Daniel H. Wilson

- Create 2 positive affirmations. Write them on Post-it notes and stick them on the bathroom mirror. (E.g. I love and accept myself.)
- Research specialists you need.
- Take a 10-30 minute walk.
- Do a 10 minute meditation.
- Visit an animal or animal shelter.
- Read 1 chapter of a book.
- Eat something healthy.
- Say your mantra out loud 3 times.
- Call a supportive friend and say your affirmations out loud 3 times.

- Make a list of everything you have survived (every surgery).
- Go to the "My Solutions" List and circle something you need for self-care.

Write about the Bonus Key #6 – Accommodation:

What can you do to accommodate yourself?

_____

_____

_____

_____

_____

_____

_____

_____

Bonus Work: Post on the FB group that you finished Day #6 of the Self-Love/ Self-Starter Challenge: write your insights.

⇒**Skim over Day #7 to see what you need to plan for.**

DAY #7
ACCOMPLISHMENT!

*"Challenges are gifts that force us to search for a
new center of gravity. Don't fight them. Just
find a new way to stand."*
—Oprah Winfrey

- Write down 10 things you are grateful for.
- Say your mantra out loud 3 times.
- Look back at your goals and reflect.
- Take a 30–60 minute walk.
- Do a 10–20 minute meditation.
- Post your affirmations by your computer and kitchen.
- Wear your new item of clothing out to an event.
- Attend a support group, therapy session, or free coaching call, or make a new friend.
- Write a thank you note. Thank a parent, friend, or doctor for helping you.
- Rearrange some furniture in your bedroom or living area.
- Visit or view some beautiful art for 15 minutes.
- Attend a performance or listen to some live music.
- Write your own Day #8 list.

Write about your progress over the past 7 days.

What have you changed, accomplished, or enjoyed?

_____

_____

_____

_____

_____

_____

_____

_____

Bonus Work: Post on the FB group that you finished Day #6 of the Self-Love/ Self-Starter Challenge: write your insights.

DO: Find some way to celebrate a full week of self-love and completing the 7-day challenge.

Remember This:

> "No one is useless in this world who lightens the
> burdens of another."
> —Charles Dickens

FROM A HIGHER PERSPECTIVE

From a higher perspective things don't look the same.
The way we see things changes
the more we move up, the farther away,
To higher realms and vantage points.

The trees become sticks,
the mountains are molehills
The craters small holes,
the burnt village a little brown blip
surrounded by teeming green life.

In the grand scheme of things,
the most major important thing before you is
just a page in a short chapter of a series of never-ending novels
Mattering only intensely to that single moment.
Then, the moment passes.

What is/was so big becomes so small
(when the camera is pulled back)
- to take all the years into account.

May we ride the small waves
May we weather the tiny drops of rain, each at a time.
May we endure the dark night, the bad day, the month-long health
crisis. . .

May we reach outside of ourselves to a higher perspective to get a full
view of the totality of the situation, predicament, problem... or the
dilemma we are dealing with.

May not one wave drown us.
May not one drop of rain engulf us.
May not one bad episode be the end all the good,
but rather the end of just that thing.

For it is only love that matters with corrected clear vision.
It is only the blessings of love that was left behind, that our Souls are
counting.
And it is the larger vantage point of love that gets us through.

-Sonya Zappone 2020

HELPFUL RESOURCES

National Suicide Prevention Hotline

https://suicidepreventionlifeline.org/
24/7 Crisis Hotline: National Suicide Prevention Lifeline Network
1-800-273-8255

American Federation of Suicide Prevention

https://afsp.org/suicide-prevention-resources

National Institute of Health

Genetic and Rare Diseases Information Center (GARD)
https://rarediseases.info.nih.gov/diseases/6322/ehlers-danlos-syndromes

Ehlers-Danlos Society

https://www.ehlers-danlos.com/
https://www.ehlers-danlos.com/eds-helpline/

Please call the Helpline at 248-716-8336. Leave a message, including the time zone that you're calling from. The Helpline staff will call you back (usually within three business days.)

Ehlers-Danlos Support UK

https://www.ehlers-danlos.org

EDS News

https://ehlersdanlosnews.com/

MCAS websites:

https://mastcellresearch.com/
https://tmsforacure.org/overview/
https://mastcell360.com/

Like this book? Please LIKE the Facebook Book Page:

EDS Survival Guide: 5 Keys to Thriving with Ehlers-Danlos Syndrome
https://www.facebook.com/EDS-Survival-Guide-5-Keys-to-Thriving-with-Ehlers-Danlos-Syndrome-109410748166516

Need a community of support? Join our Facebook Group:

EDS Surviving to Thriving Group
https://www.facebook.com/groups/164458749205702

ABOUT THE AUTHOR

*"Years may wrinkle the skin, but to give up
enthusiasm wrinkles the soul."*
—Samuel Ullman

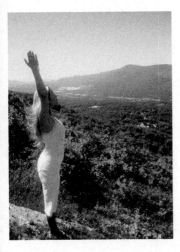

Sonya Zappone, RYT, C.MI, C.CLAC, is a certified life coach, yoga and meditation instructor, devoted mother, and author of *The Soul Doesn't Need a Million Dollars* and *Connect to Soul: Poems for Yoga.*

Dedicated to following her Soul's calling, Sonya actively encourages others to do the same by pursuing work that they love and leading their lives with light, love, and wisdom. For many years she was a cherished yoga teacher and leader of transformational workshops and retreats to strengthen, nourish, and connect attendees at the mind, body, spirit, and Soul level.

From her deep respect of the resilient body and a personal quest for healing, Sonya dedicates herself to the study, practice, and teachings of yoga. She feels incredibly grateful to have led senior chair yoga for the wise elders of her community for as long as she did. She says that she learned more from her students than any educational program could ever offer because life experience is invaluable.

After more than eleven years of instructing yoga classes in her community and designing and implementing specialized, uniquely crafted healing retreats, she has moved on to online teachings. She enjoys reaching those seeking healing through yoga and meditation. You can find Sonya's yoga videos, meditations, and relaxations on her YouTube channel, "Yoga for All of You."

Sonya draws inspiration from many disciplines, spiritual teachings, yoga instructors, and numerous authors. She spends most of her time loving and guiding her daughter through a happy childhood and dedicates the rest to writing the truth as she recognizes it, hoping to make the world a better, nicer, kinder, softer place.

Please visit her on the web at SonyaZappone.com

Made in the USA
Middletown, DE
04 October 2023